ACKNOWLEDGEMENTS

sports coach UK, St Andrew's Ambulance Association and sportscotland would like to thank the following individuals for their major contribution toward the writing of this handbook:

Mr Donald Macleod . . . . Consultant Surgeon,
St John's Hospital, Livingston

Mr Jimmy Graham . . . . Consultant Orthopedic Surgeon,
Western Infirmary, Glasgow

Dr Ian Pinkerton . . . . St Andrew's Ambulance Association

Dr Jim Junor. . . . . St Andrew's Ambulance Association

Ms Kirsty Arbuthnott. . . . . Chartered Physiotherapist,
Southern General Hospital, Glasgow

Dr Wendy Dodds . . . . Consultant Rheumatologist,
St Luke's Hospital, Bradford

Dr Colin Feltes . . . . General Practitioner,
Inverness

Mr James McKenna. . . . . Head Coach,
Great Britain Disabled Volleyball Team

Mrs Joan Watt. . . . . Chartered Physiotherapist,
Watt Physiotherapy Clinic, Tillicoultry

Their sterling work has ensured that the contents meet the requirements of the three voluntary aid organisations, St John Ambulance, St Andrew's Ambulance Association and British Red Cross, and are therefore applicable throughout the British Isles. The original illustrations were drawn by Archie Shanks and William Rudling.

The publishers would also like to thank Mrs Joan Watt and British Red Cross for their assistance in updating this handbook for the 2000 and 2001 reprint respectively. Finally, the publishers would like to thank Warwick Andrews, Martin Colclough and Andrew Walton for their valuable input into this edition.

Sports Injury

prevention and first aid management

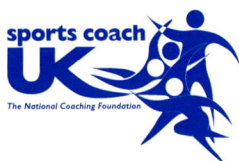

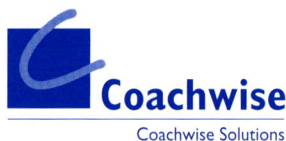

sports coach UK
114 Cardigan Road
Headingley
Leeds LS6 3BJ
Tel: 0113-274 4802 Fax: 0113-275 5019
E-mail: coaching@sportscoachuk.org
Website: www.sportscoachuk.org

Patron: HRH The Princess Royal

Published on behalf of **sports coach UK** by
Coachwise Solutions
Coachwise Ltd
Chelsea Close
Off Armley Road
Armley, Leeds LS12 4HP
Tel: 0113-231 1310 Fax: 0113-231 9606
E-mail: enquiries@coachwisesolutions.co.uk
Website: www.coachwisesolutions.co.uk

Contents

Contents

Contents

Injuries can happen when exercising or during sport. This book is for all those involved in exercise and sport – the participant, the parent, the teacher, the coach and the official. It provides a ready guide to injury prevention and first aid management. These are everyone's responsibility.

There is however, no substitute for practical training, and you should attend a recognised first aid course to supplement the advice offered in this book. As well as the more general first aid qualifications offered by St Andrew's Ambulance Association, St John Ambulance and British Red Cross, sports coach UK and British Red Cross offer an Emergency First Aid for Sport course which focuses on first aid in a sporting context. In addition, sports coach UK offers a sports injury workshop which includes first aid: Injury Prevention and Management. This handbook provides the basis of the workshop material and is presented in six main sections.

Throughout this handbook, the pronouns he, she, him, her and so on are interchangeable and intended to be inclusive of both men and women. It is important in sport, as elsewhere, that men and women have equal status and opportunities.

PUBLISHER'S WARNING

The contents of this handbook follow the International Consensus concerning First Aid Procedures. However, the publishers accept no legal liability whatsoever for any actions taken which contravene the advice and instruction given within this handbook.

The handbook can be used as a guideline for treatment by the untrained. However, the lifesaving techniques of rescue breaths and external chest compression, and the techniques for the management of spinal injuries and lifting and transporting casualties should not be used until you have received proper instructions from a qualified instructor.

Sports
Injury

INTRODUCTION

More and more people of all ages are now exercising regularly for the benefit of their health. Regular exercise is not a substitute for an unhealthy lifestyle. Being overweight, smoking, taking drugs or excess alcohol is harmful to health.

For many people exercise and sport can be fun. Everyone is different and when planning an exercise programme, age, current fitness level, aims, personal ability and time available must be considered.

If participants try to do too much too soon, they are more likely to sustain an injury. A well planned programme, combined with a sound knowledge of safe practice, will help to develop fitness and avoid injury.

Should injuries occur, prompt and appropriate treatment will minimise damage, help to achieve a quick and safe return to activity and reduce the likelihood of the injury recurring.

FIT TO PARTICIPATE?

General fitness refers to the overall physical condition of the individual and can range from illness through good health to the peak of human condition.

Fitness is affected by a number of factors – age, lifestyle, training, illness and injury, physical and psychological state, diet and rest. Individuals have considerable control over their own health and level of fitness.

A carefully planned exercise programme will readily maintain or improve an individual's general health and well-being. This might take no more than an hour a week for the average participant.

If you wish to improve your all-round fitness, the type of exercise you adopt must make your heart, lungs and muscles work hard (eg cycling, swimming, running, jogging, badminton, skipping and brisk walking). The most enjoyable way to exercise and improve your overall health, is to try to take part in one or two different sports each week. This will keep a different range of muscles and joints active, while improving the efficiency of your heart and lungs.

In addition to active exercise, you should also consider spending ten minutes a day doing exercises to improve joint flexibility and muscle strength. Remember you are never too old to benefit.

Overall fitness consists of four main components:

- Endurance (stamina)
- Strength

- Flexibility
- Speed and power.

These four components are required in varying proportions for different forms of exercise and sport. For example, cyclists need a high level of endurance, gymnasts need good strength and flexibility, sprinters need speed and strength (power).

Accordingly, it is possible to plan a training programme for any individual by blending the four main fitness components, depending on the chosen activity.

STARTING OUT

Whatever the level of participation start slowly and build up gradually.

Often people rush into a new exercise or training programme, and allow their eagerness to override their common sense. The importance of a step-by-step approach is essential. This is just as true for experienced athletes as for older participants or youngsters who are developing their fitness or sporting potential.

Any exercise programme should allow adequate time for rest and relaxation. Recuperation is an important part of training.

DIET AND SPORT

It is not necessary to have a special diet if you are involved in sport[1]. Everyone, whatever their level of activity, should eat a well balanced diet, avoiding the common error of eating too much fat and not enough carbohydrate. Carbohydrates are the main fuel supply used by muscles during activity and the best sources of this type of food are bread, pasta, potatoes and rice.

During exercise the body loses fluid through evaporation and sweat. Therefore it is essential that athletes in training and competition drink large amounts of fluid such as water or diluted fruit juice to compensate for this loss.

▶▶▶ Footnote

1   For further information on diet and sport, the **sports coach UK** Coach Workshop and resource *Fuelling Performers* are strongly recommended (see page 88).

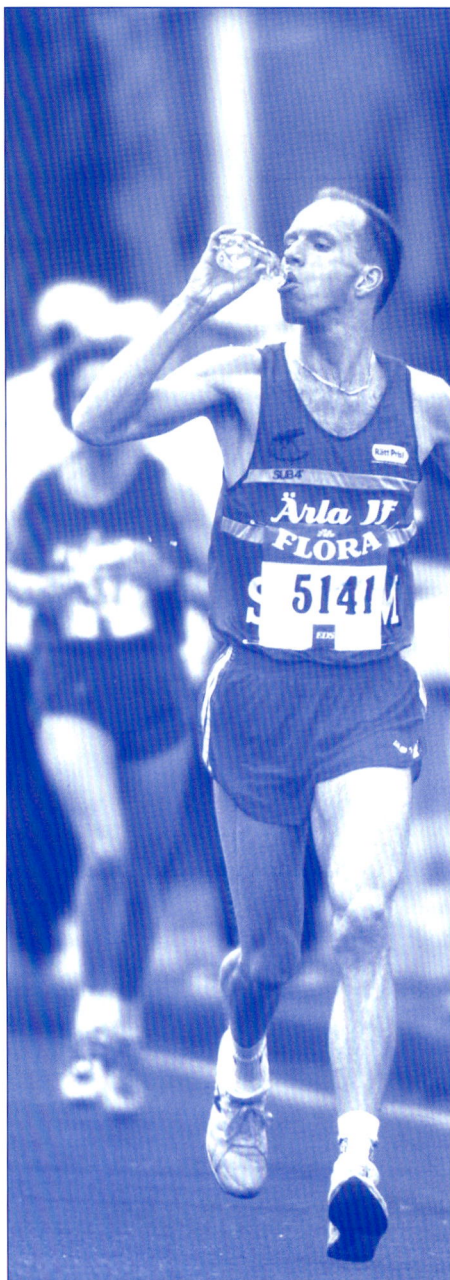

actionplus

HAZARDS IN ACTIVE EXERCISE

Active exercise can, and will, do harm in three main sets of circumstances.

First of all, too much exercise too soon in a training programme can lead to injury.

Secondly, injury or illness can occur when individuals are training vigorously, to the very limits of their capability. Under this kind of pressure the body structure can fail.

Thirdly, irrespective of the stage of the training programme, the level of fitness or the sport, injuries are more likely to occur if inappropriate, poor quality equipment is used and you do not conform to the basic rules of the activity in which you are participating. This warning particularly applies to footwear. For example, disaster will strike if you attempt to climb Ben Nevis in training shoes on a cold, wet, windy winter's day. Likewise, lower leg injuries are more likely to occur running a marathon in gym shoes rather than training shoes designed for distance running.

Section Two

2

Prevention
and
Reduction
of injuries and
illnesses in sport

CAUSES OF INJURY IN SPORT

Injuries happen in sport no matter how much care is taken and despite advances in equipment, medicine and coaching. Injuries occur most frequently in:

- high risk activities (eg downhill skiing)
- contact sports (eg rugby)
- sports making extreme demands on muscle strength (eg weightlifting).

Injuries are more likely to occur in poor conditions, (eg extremes of temperature, wind, rain and poor light). The most common injuries affect the soft tissues (skin, muscle, ligament, tendon), the bones and the joints. Less common but potentially more serious injuries can occur to the internal organs (brain, spinal cord, chest and abdominal organs).

There are two principal causes of injury:

- direct or extrinsic – as the result of a fall or blow
- indirect or intrinsic – when tissues break down or become inflamed as a result of repeated stress or overuse. The indirect injury usually results from poor technique, unsuitable equipment, inappropriate training programmes, overtraining, poor practice procedures or sudden, unexpected overload.

CAUSES OF ILLNESS IN SPORT

ENVIRONMENTAL FACTORS

Changes in environmental conditions can make inappropriately equipped people and even highly trained athletes more prone to illness.

Illnesses which can arise from changes in environmental conditions include:

- hypothermia (dangerous lowering of body temperature) from exposure to extreme cold and inclement weather (wind and rain)
- heat exhaustion from high temperatures and dehydration
- mountain sickness (oxygen reduction) at high altitudes
- the bends (nitrogen decompression sickness) from too rapid a reduction in pressure after exposure to high pressures (eg deep sea diving).

Individuals should **never** participate in vigorous exercise and sport if they have a **temperature or flu-like symptoms**. Any participant in sport (and especially veterans) must seek medical advice if undue breathlessness or chest pains develop while exercising. It is important that parents, teachers and coaches are aware of these risks.

OVERTRAINING

Overtraining will result in ill-health as well as loss of form and increased likelihood of injury. The symptoms of overtraining include listlessness, poor appetite, sleep disturbance, weight loss, loss of form and an absence of menstruation in females.

HOW CAN THE INCIDENCE OF INJURIES BE REDUCED?

The incidence of injuries can be reduced by:

- choosing a suitable programme or sport activity for the individual
- ensuring that the individual is fit to participate
- adopting appropriate safety and preventative measures
- ensuring adequate supervision and good advice
- adhering to the rules of the chosen activity.

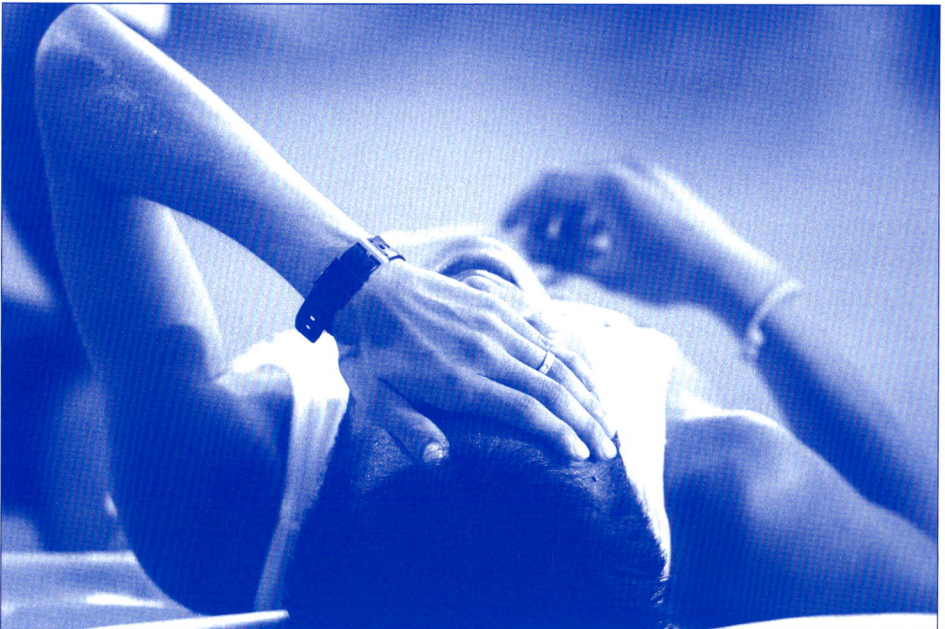

actionplus

CHOICE OF PROGRAMME ACTIVITY

Any individual embarking on a new activity, or advising others, must take many factors into consideration when selecting an appropriate programme.

PHYSICAL CHARACTERISTICS

Participation in a sport or exercise for which an individual is not well suited may increase the likelihood of injury. Certain minor physical deformities (eg flat feet) would make an individual more prone to ankle, leg or knee injuries. Therefore an activity such as long distance road running would not be advisable.

INTEREST

People take part in sport for different reasons – for the fun of it, to improve their skills, to compete against others, to win. Competitive sport can provide new challenges, increase enjoyment and may even become the prime motivation for continuing participation. Winners thrive on competition but striving for success can create psychological pressure, particularly if the competitive element is being encouraged by over-ambitious parents, teachers or coaches.

Exercise and sport should be fun and the needs and interests of the individual should always come first. Special consideration should be given to the interests of young people, women (especially expectant mothers), veterans and people with disabilities or additional needs.

CHILDREN AND YOUNG PEOPLE

Children and young people are not mini-adults. They require specially designed programmes, not scaled down adult sports or training plans. Steady, low-intensity exercise, with adequate periods of rest, is more suitable.

Although girls and boys are physically very similar before puberty, they have their peak growth rates at different ages – girls usually between 10 and 12, boys about two years later. During this growth period, their bones cannot cope with heavy or intensive training programmes. These could cause growing pains, affecting knees, heels, elbows, shoulders and the back. Specific strength and weight training should be avoided and strength developed naturally using their own body weight as a resistance (eg press-ups, pull-ups).

Providing children with good quality equipment can be expensive during this period of rapid growth and development. Growing children must be given the best quality footwear appropriate for their sport, even if this means a new pair of shoes every six to twelve months during a rapid growth spurt.

The same principle applies to the use of protective equipment such as a mouthguard which should be individually fitted for the young person by their own dentist, and changed as often as necessary.

The physical changes at puberty may result in the need for changes in technique. Girls, for example, develop a wider pelvis (to facilitate child birth) and this may affect the running action and even cause pain in the front of the knee.

In addition to physical developments, childhood and adolescence may bring emotional stresses – particularly for early and late developers. It is important to ensure that young people enjoy a variety of sport and exercise programmes, that frustration is avoided by ensuring the activity is appropriate for them (emotionally as well as physically) and that competition is kept in perspective.

Girls may be sensitive about participating in sport when they start having periods, and need reassurance that a normal period does not prevent participation in even the most vigorous activities.

WOMEN

Women may choose to regulate their periods by taking the contraceptive pill, but many find that they perform better at sport if they have a normal menstrual cycle.

Girls and women involved in very intense training programmes may find that their periods become scanty or even stop. If this occurs, the performer should consult her doctor to check there is nothing seriously wrong. In most cases, this condition will be corrected by adjusting the training programme, and gaining a little weight.

A normal pregnancy should not, as a rule, prevent physical activity, but it is important that pregnant women consult regularly with their general practitioner, or obstetrician, about the type and amount of exercise they are taking, adjusting their exercise programme accordingly. In the early months, brisk walking can help maintain fitness, but later, swimming is more appropriate (avoid breast stroke). A good exercise programme throughout pregnancy will help maintain fitness and firm muscles, at the same time controlling unnecessary weight gain, and promoting the rapid return of a slim active figure after the baby has been born.

Breast feeding does not rule out exercise, but a good supporting maternity bra is essential. It is important to choose the type of exercise carefully, as jogging would obviously be uncomfortable, whereas brisk walking, cycling and swimming would be beneficial and more comfortable.

VETERANS

There are increasing numbers of older adults becoming involved in sport and in masters events. There are some sensible guidelines that can be followed, particularly if they are just taking up or resuming sport at this age. A simple guide can be obtained by:

- consulting a doctor for a check on weight, pulse rate, blood pressure, heart, lungs, urine and blood

- reassessing lifestyle, particularly with regard to the amount of everyday exercise, dietary habits, drinking and smoking

- choosing an activity carefully, starting slowly and building up gradually – stretching exercises to maintain flexibility are particularly important for veterans.

DISABLED PEOPLE

Disabled people and those with additional needs benefit from active play, exercise or sport. Activity offers a healthier lifestyle, a feeling of well-being and the opportunity for communication and contact with other people. It can be a challenge to find the right activity to suit individual physical or psychological capability. It is advisable to consult a doctor before recommending or taking up any new activity.

The scope is wide, and advice is readily available from many organisations (see page 94).

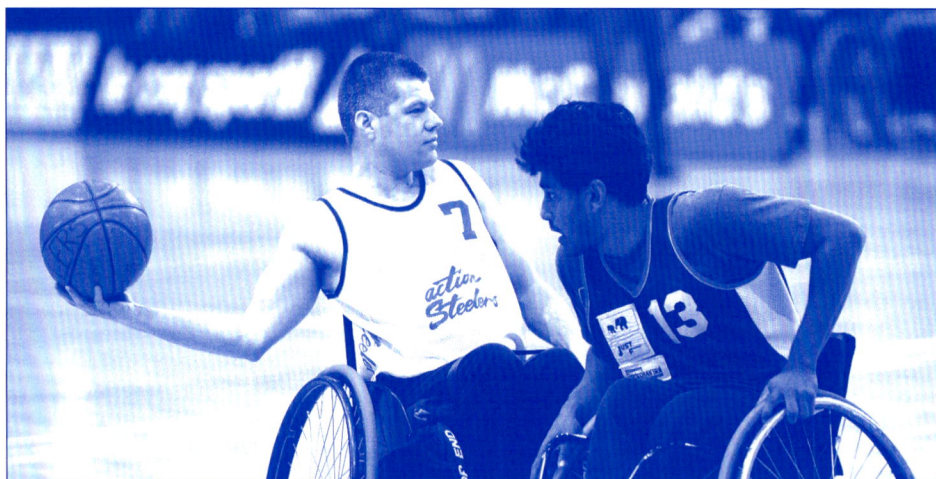

actionplus

FITNESS ASSESSMENT

If flexibility, strength, speed and endurance are inadequate for the chosen sport or activity, injuries are more likely to occur. It is important to know how to assess fitness as well as the type of fitness required for each sport.

General fitness can be gauged through health checks carried out by a doctor or less accurately through self-assessment measure (eg resting pulse rate, recovery time for return to resting rates following exercise). Athletes wishing to measure more accurately the components of fitness require either recognised field tests or a laboratory test. The latter is more costly and time-consuming and should always be carried out by specialists at registered institutions[1]. Field tests are more accessible and sometimes more appropriate for the sport. Tests have been developed to measure endurance, strength, speed and flexibility and these can generally be carried out without specialist facilities. For example, the multi-stage fitness test[2] is a progressive shuttle run test which can be undertaken in a gym, on a field or a track. It will provide an estimation of endurance fitness[3].

►►► Footnote

1   For further information on laboratory and field fitness tests, contact BASES (The British Association of Sport and Exercise Sciences), Tel: 0113-289 1020 Website: www.bases.org.uk

2   Available from Coachwise 1st4sport (Tel: 0113-201 5555 Website: www.1st4sport.com).

3   For further information on fitness testing, refer to the home study pack *A Guide to Field Based Fitness Testing* available from Coachwise 1st4sport (Tel: 0113-201 5555 Website: www.1st4sport.com).

FITNESS REQUIREMENTS

FLEXIBILITY

In all sports, some degree of flexibility (suppleness) is needed for effective performance and injury avoidance. Different muscles and tendons are at risk in different sports, and injuries will occur if a muscle is stretched beyond its normal range of movement. Regular stretching improves the elasticity of muscles and tendons. This should be carried out smoothly and under control by:

- slowly moving the muscle group concerned with a particular movement to the stretched position until discomfort (not pain) is felt
- holding the position for about 20 to 30 seconds.

Three stretches should be completed for each muscle group. Working opposing muscle groups in sequence gives best results.

NB Ensure muscle is warm before stretching. Raise body temperature by jogging or some form of similar activity.

Too much flexibility can also result in injury if there is insufficient strength to support the movement of the joint. It is equally important to maintain a balance in strength between groups of muscles that work against each other (eg between the hamstring muscles at the back of the thigh and the quadriceps at the front).

STRENGTH AND SPEED

Regain full range of movement before engaging in strength training which should be tailored to the needs of the individual, and not overdone. It is generally recommended that weights should not be used until bone development is complete (about 17 years). It should also be adapted to the activity in terms of the:

- muscles used (eg distance runners need less upper body strength work than gymnasts)
- training load (eg the gymnast needs muscle strength gained by few repetitions of moving heavy loads; the runner needs muscle endurance gained by moving light loads with more frequent repetitions).

During injury, muscle wasting often occurs and it is important that muscle strength is regained before full training is resumed. Speed of movement is important for a number of sports and specific training is needed for its development.

ENDURANCE

Endurance is required to offset fatigue which usually results in the breakdown of skill – noticeable, for example, in the loss of style in the distance runner and the technique change in the tennis player. Performance is impaired and there is an increased risk of overuse injury.

Endurance fitness must be gained slowly if it is to be achieved safely and should be specific:

- Cardiorespiratory fitness is gained by extending the body's ability to supply oxygen to the working muscle. Typically this involves exercising the large muscle groups (eg in running, swimming and cycling).

- Local muscle endurance increases the stamina of a particular muscle group (eg sit-ups will increase the endurance of the stomach muscles but will contribute little to cardiorespiratory fitness).

SAFETY AND PREVENTATIVE MEASURES

WARM-UP

Warm-up is a very important factor in the prevention of injury. It should be used not only before the start but following any breaks in activity (eg after an interval, before each routine, race or bout). It should be enjoyable, related to the activity to follow and consist of three phases:

- Full body exercises involving both arms and legs, carried out at an increasing pace (to raise body temperature and the rate of blood flow).

- Slow, sustained stretching of each of the muscles, tendons and joints to prepare them for use, working systematically through the body and paying extra attention to those muscles likely to be placed under the greatest stress.

- Skill exercises to simulate the practice or competitive conditions to prepare mentally and physically.

COOL-DOWN

Cool-down is equally important at the end of the activity. This helps the body to recover gradually and prevents the build up of fluids in the muscles which can lead to subsequent soreness and stiffness. A cool-down, which might last about 15 minutes, should consist of mild, rhythmic activity and the gentle stretching of the muscles which have been working. Warm (not hot) baths, showers or massage may also help recovery and reduce possible soreness.

SKILL

Injuries are more likely if technique is poor, if the skill level is inadequate for the situation (eg a highly skilled judo player should not compete against a novice) or where skills break down due to competitive stress or fatigue. More skilful performers are less prone to injury and less likely to cause injury.

Incorrect technique can result in overuse injuries so coaches must be able to assess and correct technique.

A breaststroke swimmer with too wide a leg kick may suffer knee injuries (in addition to producing a less efficient kick).

The acquisition of skill and good technique often takes many hours of repetitive practice which can result in overuse injuries. Skill development, like fitness, should be developed slowly and progressively.

CLOTHING, EQUIPMENT AND FACILITIES

Well designed clothing and good quality equipment are essential if accidents and injuries are to be avoided. Footwear design has advanced considerably and shoes must be appropriate to the individual, the sport and the surface.

Participation in a range of sports will require more than one pair of shoes and if the feet are still growing, frequent replacement is essential although costly.

It is important that protective clothing is used for the purpose for which it has been designed. Lacrosse helmets protect the skull from frequent impacts, cycling helmets or riding hats from a single more serious impact. Protection may be impaired following a major impact or over a long period of time – even though no damage is apparent. Mouthguards should be used in contact sports and these must be made for the individual by a dentist. Individuals wearing glasses should use shatter-proof lenses or contact lenses, as a form of eye protection in squash.

Equipment should be of good quality and purpose built. Worn-out, part serviceable or adapted equipment may cut costs but it frequently leads to accidents or injuries.

Sometimes equipment is used for a purpose for which it is not intended or is adapted to meet a different need (eg judo mats being used for gymnastics). This is inappropriate and can result in injury.

Sport and exercise should always take place in a suitable, well-maintained environment. Obviously, an uneven or slippery surface, or a potholed football pitch, will increase the risk of injury. Protection should always be found against unavoidable hazards (eg fencing, posts, windows).

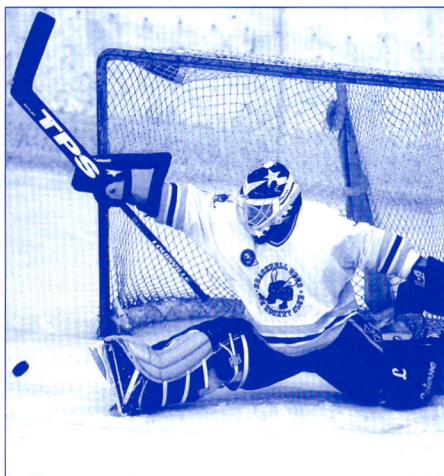

actionplus

ADEQUATE SUPERVISION

Injuries in sport occur more frequently if there is inadequate supervision or poor control. This is particularly true in sports in which there is an element of danger (eg gymnastics, water sports, javelin), where the conditions are cramped or skill level is low.

Many rules are designed to protect the safety of participants as well as to ensure fair play and an evenly balanced competition. Rules should always be respected and enforced and those in charge should provide a good role model at all times.

In addition, they should:

- be trained in first aid
- become appropriately trained in the activity (eg by the governing body of sport)
- plan the activities with safety in mind
- maintain discipline
- place themselves so that all participants are in view
- use well rehearsed safety calls (eg stop signals in a swimming pool)
- check the environment for hazards before and during the activity (eg lighting, surfaces, equipment)
- ensure that equipment is regularly checked and maintained
- ensure first aid equipment is readily available at all times.

Section Three

3

Injuries
and
Illnesses
in sport

AIMS OF FIRST AIDERS IN SPORT

The aims of first aiders in sport are to:

- provide immediate care to minimise serious consequences of injury or illness

- promote recovery

- encourage measures to prevent injury.

▶▶ ACTION

- Use your head before your hands.

▶ STAY COOL

To stay cool and reassure an injured participant, you need a basic knowledge of relevant first aid which will help you adopt a systematic and reassuring approach to the injured participant.

▶ LOOK

- at the situation – is there any further danger?

- at the patient – is the patient conscious, breathing normally, bleeding, is colour normal, is the injured part obviously deformed?

▶ LISTEN

- to the patient and to any witnesses. What happened?

- Is the patient talking and answering questions sensibly?

- Does the patient know what is happening?

- Is there any dizziness or blurred vision?

▶ ASK

- the patient to try very gently to move the injured part(s) (except when dealing with any potential head or neck injury).

▶ TOUCH

- Having used your head to get a good idea of what happened to the patient, you can now use your hands to examine the injured part, comparing it to the other side of the body, head or limb.

IT IS IMPORTANT THAT NO FOOD OR DRINK IS GIVEN TO ANY INJURED PERFORMER WHO MAY REQUIRE HOSPITAL TREATMENT.

THE ABC OF RESUSCITATION

AIRWAY

- In all unconscious casualties, a clear airway to the lungs is essential.

- Open the airway by placing one hand on the forehead, gently tilting the head back and lifing the chin.

- Remove any obvious obstructions from the mouth (eg gumshield).

BREATHING

- Check if the casualty is breathing.

- Kneel down beside the casualty and place your cheek as near to his mouth as possible (see Figure 1). Look, listen and feel for any signs of breathing for up to ten seconds.

Figure 1

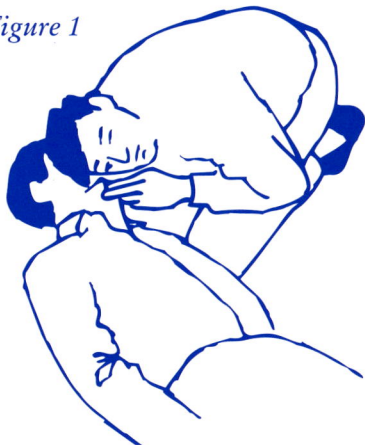

CIRCULATION

- Look for signs of circulation, such as movement, breathing, coughing or normal skin colour, for up to ten seconds.

Figure 2

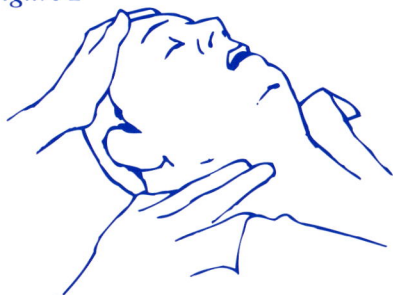

RESCUE BREATHS

If the casualty is not breathing but circulation is present, give rescue breaths:

1 Keep the airway open by head tilt and chin support.

2 Pinch the casualty's nose with the fingers and thumb of one hand.

3 Take a deep breath, open your mouth and seal your lips completely over the casualty's mouth (see Figure 3). Blow firmly and steadily until you see the chest rise.

Figure 3

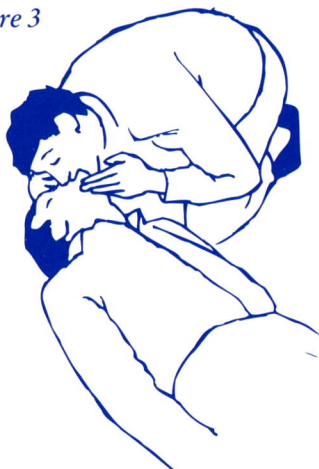

4 Lift your mouth away from the casualty's mouth and turn your head towards his chest. If the rescue breath has been successful, you will be able to see his chest falling as the air comes out of the lungs. Aim for a rate of one breath every six seconds.

5 Repeat Steps 1 to 4.

6 After giving two breaths, check for signs of circulation (eg movement, breathing, coughing, normal skin colour) for up to ten seconds.

7 If circulation is present, give ten rescue breaths in a minute. If circulation is absent, or you are at all unsure, commence CPR immediately (see below).

8 Continue rescue breaths until help arrives. Check circulation after every minute. If circulation stops at any stage, commence CPR.

9 If breathing returns, turn the casualty into the recovery position (see page 22) and monitor breathing and pulse until help arrives.

CARDIOPULMONARY RESUSCITATION (CPR)

(FOR ADULTS AND CHILDREN AGED EIGHT YEARS AND OVER)

1 Kneel on the casualty's left or right side. Place the middle finger of your lower hand on the point where his ribs meet and the index finger above.

2 Put the heel of your other hand on the breastbone next to the fingers (Figure 4). This is the point where you will apply pressure.

Figure 4

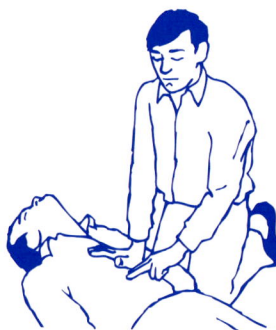

3 Cover the upper hand with the heel of your other hand and then lock your fingers together.

4 Kneel upright with your shoulders over the casualty's breastbone. Keep your arms straight. Give 15 chest compressions – for each compression, press down about 4–5cm or $1/_2$–2 inches. Release the pressure, but do not remove your hands from the chest.

5 After giving 15 chest compressions, tilt the casualty's head back, lift his chin and give two rescue breaths (see page 19). Continue this cycle of chest compressions and breaths until help arrives. If there are signs of recovery, check airway, breathing and circulation again.

IMPORTANT

No harm will be done to the casualty if rescue breaths are given and the casualty is still breathing, but chest compression may be dangerous if performed when the heart is beating even feebly. Therefore chest compression must not be given unless the signs of failure of circulation are positively identified:

- casualty is unconscious
- there is no breathing
- there are no signs of circulation.

When performing chest compression, the casualty must be on a firm surface. The pressure must be by the heel of the hand only and directed to the breast bone only – not onto the front of the ribs. Excessive pressure will cause internal injury.

It is rare for children's hearts to stop; if chest compression is necessary:

- put the heel of just one hand on the chest as for an adult
- press down five times – for each compression, press down about a third of the depth of the chest
- give one rescue breath
- continue this for one minute and then call an ambulance
- continue to give CPR until help arrives.

RECOVERY POSITION

The recovery position is used for the unconscious casualty who is breathing, or where in a conscious casualty there is a risk of airway obstruction due to vomiting or injury.

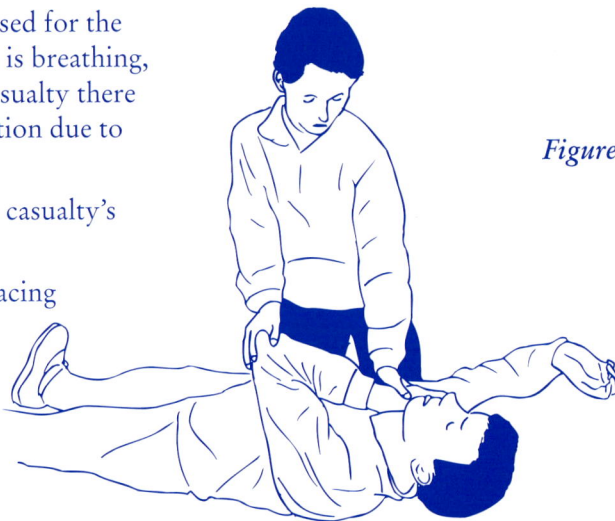

Figure 5

- Kneel facing across the casualty's chest.

- Open the airway by placing one hand on the forehead, gently tilting the head back and lifting the chin.

- Straighten the casualty's legs.

- Place nearer arm at right angles to his trunk, with elbow bent and palm of hand up.

- Bring his other arm across his chest and hold the hand, palm outwards, against his near cheek (Figure 5).

- With your other hand grasp his far thigh just above the knee. Lift the knee up, leaving the foot flat on the ground. Pull with this hand to roll the casualty towards you onto his side, while supporting his head with his hand against his cheek with your other hand (Figure 6).

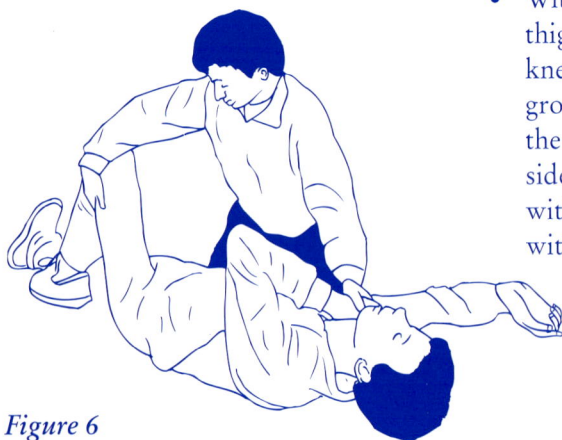

Figure 6

- Gently remove your hand from under his head and tilt his head back to keep the airway open.
- Pull the knee of the upper leg forward so that the limb is bent at the hip and knee at a right angle to support the lower body (Figure 7).

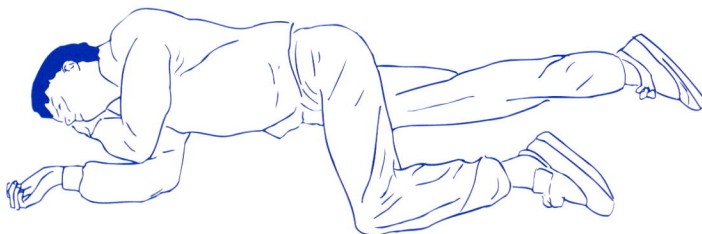

Figure 7

- Check the final position is stable; ensure that the head remains tilted with the lower jaw forward to maintain the open airway (Figure 8). If necessary, adjust the hand under his cheek.
- Call an ambulance.
- Check breathing and circulation at regular, frequent intervals.

IMPORTANT

If a spinal injury is suspected, the greatest possible care must be taken to place the casualty in the recovery position.

Ideally the procedure should be modified to ensure the head, neck and trunk are kept in alignment throughout the manoeuvre. Helpers should be used if available.

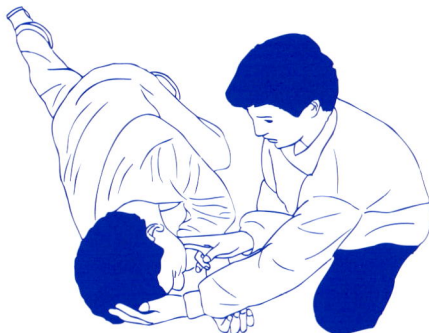

Figure 8

BLEEDING

To operate efficiently, the body has to have enough blood circulating at sufficient pressure to maintain delivery of nutriment and oxygen to all the body tissues. Severe blood loss in sport is unusual, but where it does occur, whether external or internal, it reduces the circulation and may result in the death of the casualty.

CHECKLIST FOR INITIAL ASSESSMENT

- Is the bleeding profuse? Is the blood spurting? Flowing briskly? Are major blood vessels involved?

- Does the casualty show symptoms and signs of shock (eg paleness, lightheadedness, nausea, cold, thirst, reduced level of consciousness)?

▶▶ ACTION

- If possible wash your hands thoroughly before treating casualty.

- If available, wear disposable gloves. Alternatively, cover your hands with clean plastic bags.

- Cover wound with clean pad if available and apply hand pressure. If pad is not available, ask casualty to press on wound with own hand or fingers (if capable).

If not, use your hand to apply pressure to keep edges of wound together.

- Lie casualty down with head kept low.

- Raise the part which is bleeding as high above the chest as possible.

- Apply sterile dressing and bandage firmly in position.

- Keep part raised and supported to prevent movement, and obtain medical assistance.

- If bleeding continues apply further pressure to dressing by padding and firmer bandage, or with your hand. Do not remove dressing already applied. Raise part further if possible.

- Minimise contact with shed blood and wash hands as soon as possible after treatment.

FOLLOW-UP ADVICE

All wounds which have bled profusely should be seen by a doctor, as medical treatment is likely to be required to prevent later complications.

SHOCK

Shock is a condition in which the circulation fails because either the pressure or volume of circulating blood has fallen to a dangerous level and is insufficient to maintain normal function of the vital organs. The volume of blood in circulation may be reduced as a result of internal or external bleeding or burns. The blood pressure may also fall in sudden illness (eg a heart attack). Other factors may result in a temporary reduction in blood pressure leading to a faint.

CHECKLIST FOR INITIAL ASSESSMENT

- Note colour of face, particularly areas normally pink in colour, (eg inside of lips – have they become pale?).

- Enquire for lightheadedness, nausea, cold or thirst.

- Observe circulation and breathing. Rapid, weak pulse and shallow breathing with yawning or sighing are signs of shock.

- Feel the skin – cold clammy skin is a sign of shock.

▶▶ACTION

- Treat any obvious injuries, such as bleeding, burns or broken bones.

- Lie casualty down with head low; raise and support legs if possible.

- Loosen any tight clothing, particularly around chest, waist and neck.

- Protect from cold (put something under the casualty if ground is damp). If possible, transport to nearby shelter on a stretcher.

- Dial 999 for ambulance.

- Reassure with encouraging words.

- **Do not give anything to drink or eat.** The mouth may be moistened to help relieve thirst, but drinking or eating can be dangerous.

- Check the casualty's breathing, circulation and level of response at regular intervals.

FOLLOW-UP ADVICE

After recovery, strenuous exercise should be avoided for some time and activity built up gradually with medical approval.

UNCONSCIOUSNESS

Unconsciousness results from disturbance of the function of the brain. This may arise from head injury or from interference with the blood circulation to the brain. Reduction of blood flow to the brain may be temporary as in fainting, or more permanent as in heart attack or stroke. There are also other conditions which may affect the working of the brain, but irrespective of the cause of unconsciousness the casualty has three vital needs:

A airway which is open and clear

B adequate breathing

C sufficient circulation.

CHECKLIST FOR INITIAL ASSESSMENT

Speak to and touch casualty:
• Is there any response?

Do the eyes open:
• spontaneously?
• on being spoken to?
• on painful stimulus?

Does the casualty speak:
• normally?
• is there confusion?

Does the casualty move:
• spontaneously?
• on command?
• on painful stimulus?

▶▶ ACTION

If no initial response, follow the ABC of resuscitation (see page 19) to assess whether the casualty is breathing and whether circulation is present.

If the casualty is:
• **breathing,** follow the procedures in the first column on page 27
• **not breathing,** follow the procedures in the second column on page 27
• **not breathing and circulation is absent,** follow the procedures in the third column on page 27.

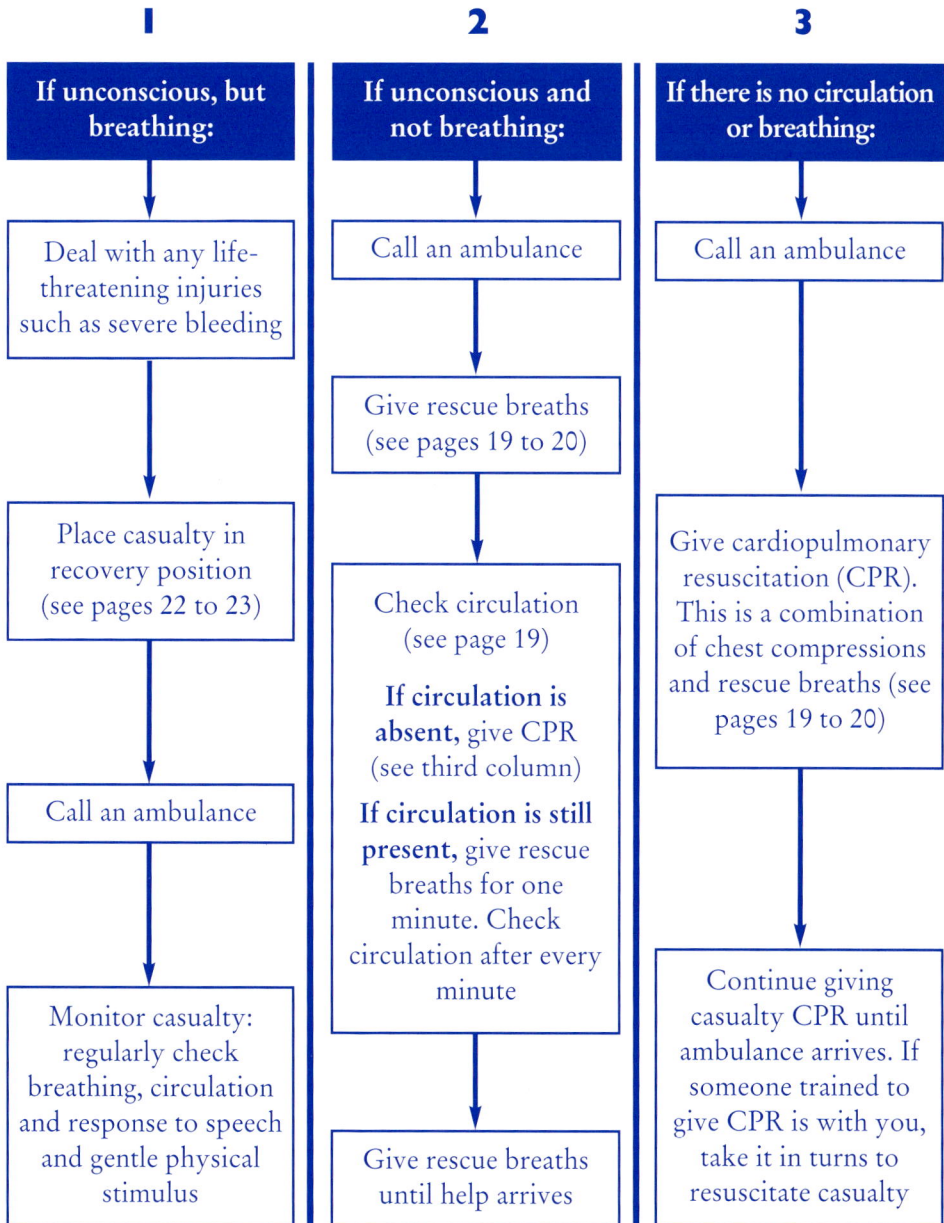

1

If unconscious, but breathing:

↓

Deal with any life-threatening injuries such as severe bleeding

↓

Place casualty in recovery position (see pages 22 to 23)

↓

Call an ambulance

↓

Monitor casualty: regularly check breathing, circulation and response to speech and gentle physical stimulus

2

If unconscious and not breathing:

↓

Call an ambulance

↓

Give rescue breaths (see pages 19 to 20)

↓

Check circulation (see page 19) **If circulation is absent,** give CPR (see third column) **If circulation is still present,** give rescue breaths for one minute. Check circulation after every minute

↓

Give rescue breaths until help arrives

3

If there is no circulation or breathing:

↓

Call an ambulance

↓

Give cardiopulmonary resuscitation (CPR). This is a combination of chest compressions and rescue breaths (see pages 19 to 20)

↓

Continue giving casualty CPR until ambulance arrives. If someone trained to give CPR is with you, take it in turns to resuscitate casualty

COLD EXPOSURE

HYPOTHERMIA

Hypothermia develops when the body temperature drops below 35°C (95°F). This condition is caused when taking part in an activity in chilling conditions (eg cold, wet, windy weather) or immersion in cold water, and is aggravated by drinking alcohol. Hypothermia can occur particularly in unfit individuals when they become tired and slow down.

To minimise the risk of suffering from hypothermia, plan and train for the activity, recognising the possibility of adverse weather conditions and having due regard to the capabilities of the participants. Wear appropriate clothing with an outer waterproof layer providing the best protection. Carry spare dry clothing, a survival bag and take high energy foods.

CHECKLIST FOR INITIAL ASSESSMENT

- Is the casualty's skin pale and very cold?

- Is the casualty shivering?

- Is the casualty forgetful, confused, clumsy, lethargic (eg stumbling or short tempered)?

- Is the casualty's breathing slow and the pulse weak?

▶▶ ACTION

- Do not continue activity which has caused hypothermia.

- Provide shelter from chilling conditions.

- If possible, replace wet clothing with dry clothing as soon as possible.

- If the casualty is young and fit he can be rewarmed by taking a bath. The water temperature should be 40°C (104°F).

- It is important that casualty should be kept dry and insulated from cold and dampness, including the ground, using sleeping bag, blankets or survival bag.

- If possible, give warm drinks and high energy foods if conscious and able to swallow.

- Individuals unaffected by the conditions should be sent for help to evacuate casualty by stretcher.

- Do not leave casualty alone unless absolutely necessary.

- Call a doctor.

Note: When the core temperature drops below about 33°C, shivering stops.

FROSTBITE

This is a condition where extreme cold causes tissue damage in the extremities (eg fingers, toes, ears, nose and cheeks).

To minimise the risk of frostbite, wear adequate boots, mittens and cover the skin of the face as much as possible.

CHECKLIST FOR INITIAL ASSESSMENT

- Has the casualty been exposed to freezing temperatures?
- Has the casualty complained of tingling and pain followed by numbness?
- Is the affected area pale, mottled blue or black in colour?

▶▶ACTION

- Handle the affected part gently. Do not rub.
- Warm the affected area slowly and naturally with continuing protection against cold.
- Arrange removal to hospital.

EFFECTS OF OVERHEATING

HEAT EXHAUSTION

This condition is caused by failure to maintain an adequate intake of fluid or to replace lost fluid and salt from the body when undertaking activities (especially endurance events) in hot, humid conditions.

Other causes of fluid loss (eg vomiting or diarrhoea) will aggravate the condition.

CHECKLIST FOR INITIAL ASSESSMENT

- Are prevailing conditions likely to lead to heat exhaustion?
- Is the casualty feeling sick, thirsty, lightheaded?
- Is the casualty sweating?
- Are there muscle cramps?

▶▶ACTION

- Lie casualty down in cool shade.
- If conscious and able to swallow, give water or flavoured squashes to drink, to which about 0.5 teaspoonful of salt per 0.5 litre (1 pint) has been added.
- If symptoms persist seek medical advice.

FOLLOW-UP ADVICE

- Rest and drink plenty of fluids.
- Do not undertake strenuous activity for at least two hours.

HEATSTROKE

If in hot conditions or in certain illnesses, the body cannot control its temperature by sweating, the body temperature will rise. Above 40°C confusion, seizures and unconsciousness may develop.

CHECKLIST FOR INITIAL ASSESSMENT

- Are prevailing conditions likely to lead to heatstroke?

- Is the casualty hot and flushed?

- Is the casualty unconscious/confused?

- Is the pulse fast and strong?

- Does the casualty have a headache and feel dizzy?

▶▶ ACTION

- If unconscious, open airway, check breathing and circulation for up to ten seconds. Resuscitate if necessary and place in recovery position.

- Lay casualty down in cool place and remove their clothes. If available, wrap casualty in a cold, wet sheet and keep it wet, or sponge body down with cold or tepid water.

- Fan casualty until body temperature falls to 38°C (100.4°F) under tongue or 37.5°C (99.5°F) under armpit.

- When casualty's temperature has fallen to safe level, replace wet sheet with dry one.

- Dial 999 for ambulance.

- Regularly monitor casualty until help arrives.

ACCLIMATISATION

The effects of overheating may be precipitated by inadequate acclimatisation. Depending on such factors as the distance travelled, the resultant fatigue, temperature and humidity and altitude, a sportsperson may need several days to acclimatise before being ready to compete. Training has to be very carefully controlled, especially during the first few days.

IMPORTANT:

Anyone who collapses in an endurance event should have a rectal temperature taken if possible.

DROWNING

Remember, anyone rescued from immersion in water[1] may be suffering as a result of cold, as well as the effect of inhaling water.

CHECKLIST FOR INITIAL ASSESSMENT

- Is the casualty conscious?

- If not conscious, is casualty breathing?

- Do the circumstances indicate possible injury (eg diving into shallow water)?

- How cold is the casualty?

▶▶ ACTION

- If the casualty is unconscious and not obviously breathing, remove obvious obstructions from mouth and throat and begin rescue breaths immediately – even before removing casualty from the water if possible.

- If there is no reason to suspect a neck or spinal injury, remove casualty from water immediately. If possible, lie casualty with head down a slope (eg if on a beach).

- If a neck or spinal injury is suspected, support casualty horizontally (eg on a board), float to shallow water if possible, with head in line with trunk, and lift out of water horizontally with good support. If possible, lie casualty with head down a slope (eg if on a beach).

- Do not waste time trying to drain water from the lungs.

- Open the airway, check breathing and circulation for up to ten seconds. Resuscitate as required.

- Do not stop resuscitation until patient is warm, as hypothermia casualties may take longer to respond.

- When warm and breathing spontaneously, place casualty in recovery position even if not unconscious, as vomiting is likely.

- Remove wet clothing and dry casualty as quickly as possible. Wrap in warm dry blankets or clothing. Treat hypothermia as appropriate.

- All casualties who may have inhaled water should be removed to hospital to ensure there is no lung damage.

▶▶▶ Footnote

1 For further information contact the Royal Life Saving Society UK (see page 93).

BENDS (DECOMPRESSION SICKNESS)

After diving at length using self contained underwater breathing apparatus (SCUBA), rapid return to the surface may result in bubbles of nitrogen being formed in the tissues. This produces the symptoms and signs of decompression sickness, which is very serious and may be fatal.

CHECKLIST FOR INITIAL ASSESSMENT

- After a dive are there transient aches, itching or a rash?
- Is there pain at joints, resulting in incapacity?
- Is there any difficulty or pain in breathing?
- Is there any paralysis or loss of sensation?

▶▶ ACTION

- Lie casualty down in recovery position and arrange urgent medical help.
- Removal to hospital or other centre with decompression facilities will probably be required.

ASTHMA

This is a condition in which breathing becomes distressingly difficult. The muscles in the air passages go into spasm, causing narrowing so that it is difficult for air to flow from the air spaces in the lungs. The spasm can be caused by allergy (eg dust, animals, pollution), nervous stress or exercise. Exercise-induced asthma is believed to be caused by the cooling and drying of the airways which can occur after exercise in certain conditions. *Post-exercise airway constriction* is perhaps a better name for the condition since the effects are not fully evident until about 15 minutes after exercise.

Most people who have asthma use a blue reliever inhaler to treat themselves during an attack. However, you can also help by reassuring the casualty, thus easing an attack.

CHECKLIST FOR INITIAL ASSESSMENT

- Has the casualty difficulty in breathing (particularly breathing out)?

- Is there a history of asthma?

- Does the casualty have a wheezy cough?

- Do the casualty's face and lips have a bluish tinge?

- Is the casualty anxious and showing signs of distress?

- Does the casualty have medication (usually a blue reliever inhaler)?

▶▶ACTION

- Remain calm and reassure casualty. They will probably have blue inhaler, which should relieve attack within a few minutes.

- Help casualty to relax in position they find most comfortable (usually sitting position).

- If attack is mild and over within ten minutes, advise casualty to take second dose of inhaler and to consult own doctor.

- Dial 999 for ambulance if attack is severe and casualty shows no signs of relief from inhaler after ten minutes, or does not have inhaler, is becoming increasingly tired, or if this is first attack. While waiting for ambulance, help casualty to take second dose of inhaler, monitor breathing and circulation, and reassure them.

HYPOGLYCAEMIA

When the sugar level of the blood falls below the normal level, brain function is affected and the level of consciousness may deteriorate rapidly. This condition can occur in sports participants engaged in strenuous activity, but most commonly occurs in people suffering from diabetes controlled by insulin or drugs. The condition can occur if too much insulin is injected, a meal is missed (or there is insufficient carbohydrate), or if prolonged, strenuous or unusual exercise is taken without adjusting diet and insulin.

CHECKLIST FOR INITIAL ASSESSMENT

- Is the casualty diabetic (look for *Medicalert* bracelet/syringe/tablets)?

- Is there evidence of a hypo attack (eg cold, clammy, pale skin, trembling, dizziness, nausea, blurred vision, staggering, bad temper, tingling of lips and mouth, hunger, confusion, shallow breathing)?

- Has food been missed or is it late?

- Has there been unusual, prolonged or strenuous exercise?

▶▶ ACTION

- If hypoglycaemia is suspected, sit casualty down and give sugary drink or food (eg sugar lump, chocolate).

- Reassess the casualty.

- If there is improvement, give further sweet drinks/food and allow to rest. Advise casualty to consult their own doctor.

- If there is no improvement, treat for shock (see page 25).

- If there is no improvement, seek medical help.

- If unconscious, place in recovery position, check airway, breathing and circulation, and resuscitate as appropriate. Call an ambulance.

SEIZURES

People with epilepsy may occasionally have a seizure. There may be a brief warning of an impending seizure but they may suddenly fall and lose consciousness, become rigid with the face and neck turning bluish and congested as breathing temporarily ceases. Twitching movements follow during which breathing may become noisy with frothy saliva at the mouth. The casualty may be incontinent. Shortly afterwards, the muscles relax as consciousness is regained. There may be a period of confusion or strange behaviour before full recovery.

CHECKLIST FOR INITIAL ASSESSMENT

- Is the casualty epileptic?
- Are the signs similar to those described above?

▶▶ACTION

- Give the casualty space and protect from injury (eg move equipment, keep people back).

- Protect the head with soft padding if possible.

- If possible, loosen any tight clothing – do this very carefully as it is easy to frighten a semi-conscious person.

- Do not attempt to restrict movement or place anything in the mouth.

- When the seizure stops, open airway, check breathing and place the casualty in the recovery position.

- Remain with casualty until sure they have completely recovered and can get home.

- If the casualty knows about the condition and there is only one seizure, simply advise to consult a doctor.

- Dial 999 for an ambulance if:
  – the seizure lasts for more than ten minutes
  – unconsciousness lasts for more than ten minutes
  – consciousness is not regained between seizures
  – this is casualty's first seizure.

SOFT TISSUE INJURIES

CUTS AND GRAZES

CHECKLIST FOR INITIAL ASSESSMENT

- Is blood flowing from the wound?
- Is there dirt in or around the wound?
- Is there any associated loss of function?

▶▶ACTION

- Control bleeding (see page 24).
- If bleeding is not severe:

1 Wash your hands (if possible) before treating the wound, and wear disposable gloves (if available).

2 Sit casualty down and raise injured part.

3 Wash wound thoroughly with cold running water if available.

4 Using sterile gauze swabs, gently clean around the wound. Always work from the wound outwards and use a fresh gauze swab for each stroke.

5 Carefully remove any loose foreign objects from or around wound such as glass, metal or gravel.

6 Gently dry area around wound with gauze swab. Be careful not to disturb wound.

7 Cover area with suitable dressing:
   - Plaster for a small cut or graze
   - Sterile dressing and bandage for larger cut or graze.

8 Wash your hands as soon as possible after treating wound.

9 Rest the injured part and, if possible, keep it raised.

FOLLOW-UP ADVICE

If tetanus immunisation is not up to date suggest that this is now done.

However, if the casualty has had five tetanus immunisations in her lifetime, a booster will only be needed if the wound is likely to be infected.

If you have not been able to clean the wound thoroughly seek medical advice. Increasing pain in the wound or swelling and redness developing later may indicate infection of the wound. Advise the casualty to seek medical aid should this occur.

BRUISES AND INFLAMMATION

CHECKLIST FOR INITIAL ASSESSMENT

- Has the force applied been sufficient to cause internal injury?
- Is there any loss of function of the part?
- Is there any tenderness on the bone in the area?
- Are there symptoms or signs of shock (see page 25)?
- Are there symptoms and signs of inflammation?

SIGNS AND SYMPTOMS OF INFLAMMATION

- Redness
- Heat
- Swelling
- Pain
- Loss of function

▶▶ACTION

- If the answer to any of the above questions is *yes*, suspect more serious injury and treat appropriately.
- If in doubt about severity of injury, seek medical advice.
- Otherwise apply cold pad or ice pack (remember to place cloth between ice and skin).
- Otherwise, support injured part in comfortable position. Apply a sling if appropriate.

FOLLOW-UP ADVICE

If pain persists or any disability develops, seek medical advice.

INJURIES TO MUSCLES, LIGAMENTS AND TENDONS

Muscles consist of thousands of fibres bound together within a sheath of connective tissue.

When the muscle fibres are overstretched or torn, a **strain** results.

Tendons are cords of tissue which connect muscle to bone to enable muscles to move bones at joints. These tendons may become inflamed (tendinitis) or torn (eg rupture of Achilles Tendon). Some tendons pass through a sheath which is lined with synovial membrane, which can become inflamed (tenosynovitis).

Ligaments are made up of fibrous tissue which hold bones together at joints. These ligaments may be overstretched or torn (eg by wrenching of a joint), resulting in a **sprain**.

CHECKLIST FOR INITIAL ASSESSMENT

- How did the injury occur? Were the forces involved severe?
- Is there significant loss of function of the part?
- Is there tenderness over the bone in the area?
- Is there any deformity of the part?
- Are there symptoms and signs of shock (see page 25).

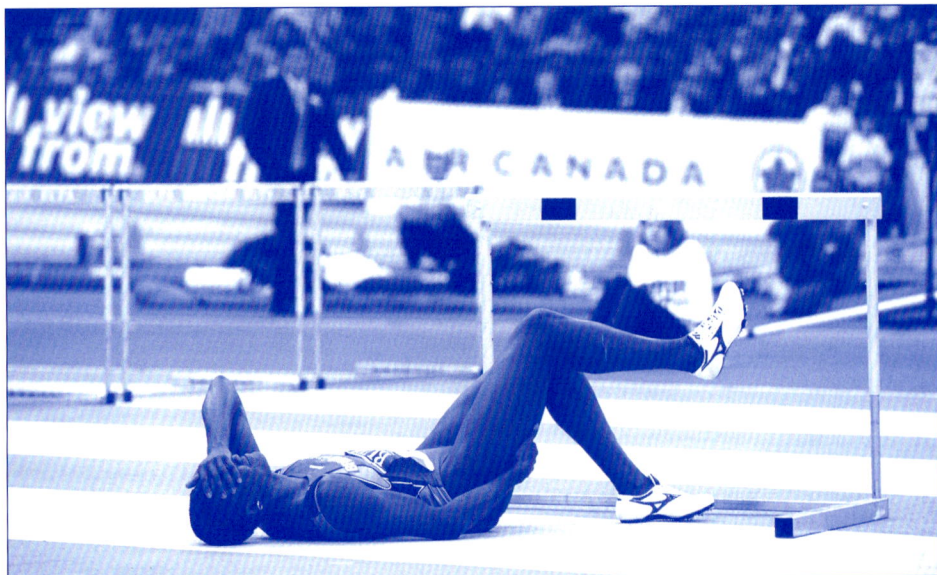

actionplus

▶▶ ACTION

- If the answer to any of these questions is *yes*, suspect more serious injury and treat as fracture (see page 40).

- If in doubt, seek medical advice.

- Otherwise, sit or lay casualty down and rest and support the part in the most comfortable position.

- Apply an ice pack or cold pad to the part for about 30 minutes.

- Apply gentle pressure by compressing injury with soft padding or securing compress with bandage.

- Raise and support injured limb to minimise bruising. If injury is to casualty's wrist, elbow or shoulder, support affected area with arm sling.

Remember the **RICE** procedure:

Rest
Ice
Compress
Elevate

FOLLOW-UP ADVICE

Keep the part rested for 24 to 72 hours before gently exercising within the limits of pain, gradually increasing the exercise daily until full fitness is restored. If pain persists or disability develops, seek medical advice. Early treatment from a chartered physiotherapist will accelerate recovery.

INJURIES TO BONES AND JOINTS

Even if moderate force is applied to the bones and joints of the body, bones can be cracked or broken (fracture) or bones can be displaced at a joint (dislocation).

CHECKLIST FOR INITIAL ASSESSMENT

- Did the casualty feel or hear a snap?
- Is there difficulty in moving the part normally?
- Is there any tenderness over a bone or joint?
- Is there deformity of the part?
- Are there symptoms and signs of shock (see page 25)?
- Is there a wound associated with the site of injury?

▶▶ACTION

- If the answer to any of these questions is *yes*, assume a significant injury.
- Steady and support the injured part in the position found, placing your hands above and below point of injury.
- Loosely cover any wound with a suitable sterile dressing.
- Do **not** attempt to replace dislocated joint to normal position.
- If the casualty has a broken arm, ask her to support it with her uninjured arm.
- Dial 999 for ambulance.
- Treat shock (see page 25) but do not raise injured limb as this causes pain.

HEAD INJURY

Head injuries can result in damage to, or disturbance of, the brain. If this occurs, then concussion or compression may result and consciousness may be clouded or lost.

CONCUSSION

This is a condition of widespread but temporary disturbance of the brain sometimes described as brain shaking. It can result from a blow to the head, a fall from a height on to the feet or a blow on the point of the jaw.

In some cases unconsciousness may have been so brief that the casualty may be unaware of, or have forgotten, the initial incident. However, because concussion can precede brain compression, it is important to observe the casualty closely after any incident involving injury to the head.

The sporting participant should be advised to stop activity for assessment and possible medical advice.

COMPRESSION OF THE BRAIN

A serious condition produced by blood accumulating within the skull or by pressure from bone in a depressed fracture. Compression may develop at any time after apparent recovery from head injury.

CHECKLIST FOR INITIAL ASSESSMENT

Level of responsiveness – including assessment of eyes, speech, understanding and movement (see page 26).

IF UNCONSCIOUS

- Is casualty breathing?
- Is breathing noisy?

▶▶ ACTION
IF UNCONSCIOUS

- Check breathing for ten seconds.
- If breathing:
  - place casualty in recovery position and ensure airway remains open
  - monitor and record casualty's condition (breathing and pulse).
- If not breathing, carry out resuscitation procedures (see pages 19–20).
- Call an ambulance if:
  - no breathing or circulation
  - casualty is unconscious for more than three minutes
  - the casualty is a child.

IF CONSCIOUS

- Check memory for recent event (eg game score) and assess eyes, speech and movement (see page 18).

- Enquire for symptoms of headache, nausea or tiredness.

- If casualty has any of the symptoms, advise them to seek medical advice.

- For less severe injuries with early apparent recovery, continue supervision and do not allow to drive or take alcohol.

CHECKLIST FOR ONGOING ASSESSMENT

- Deterioration of level of responsiveness (see page 26). Look for confusion, drowsiness, loss of coordination or seizures.

- Headache and/or vomiting?

- Slow bounding pulse?

- Pupils unequal?

▶▶ ACTION

- Dial 999 for ambulance if complications develop.

FOLLOW-UP ADVICE

Do not allow anyone with concussion or who has been knocked out, to participate in vigorous exercise or contact sport for two to four weeks, or combat sport for four to six weeks.

Anyone who is confused or knocked out for a second time within three months of their initial injury should then avoid contact or combat sport for a minimum of a further three months.

Anyone who has three concussions/knockouts in a year should rest for a year or change to a non-contact sport.

After prolonged unconsciousness in hospital or brain surgery, sporting activity should only be resumed after medical advice.

FACIAL INJURIES

Individually made and fitted mouth guards should be worn in activities where there is danger of facial injury. Injury to the face may be associated with damage to the brain or neck. The main danger is choking because the airway may become obstructed by displaced teeth, blood or saliva when the casualty is unable to swallow adequately to keep the airway clear.

CHECKLIST FOR INITIAL ASSESSMENT

- Is the casualty breathing satisfactorily?

- Is there bleeding from nose, mouth or skin?

- Is there difficulty in speaking or swallowing?

- Is there any deformity?

- Is there any disturbance of vision?

▶▶ ACTION

- Clear the mouth of any loose material (eg dentures).

- Position casualty to ensure airway is kept clear:

  – sitting – leaning forward

  – lying – in recovery position.

- Control bleeding and cover wounds.

- Obtain medical assistance.

- If teeth are partially dislocated but still attached to the gum margin, try gently to return them to the normal position. If a tooth has been knocked out and is intact with its root attached, ask the casualty to clean it by gently licking and sucking. Then ask the casualty to place it either in the socket, in the mouth between cheek and gum or in a glass of milk or water. Arrange immediate dental care.

NOSE BLEEDING

- Sit the casualty with head well forward.
- Loosen any tight clothing around the neck and chest.
- Tell casualty to pinch nostrils firmly at soft part of nose for ten minutes (Figure 9) and to breathe through the mouth. If bleeding continues, reapply pressure.
- Advise casualty to spit out any blood in mouth.
- Advise not to blow or pick nose for some time afterwards.
- If bleeding has not stopped after half an hour of continuous pressure, dial 999 for ambulance.

Note: Nose plugs should not be used.

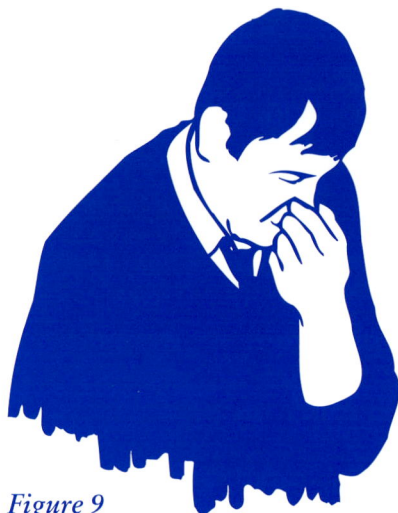

Figure 9

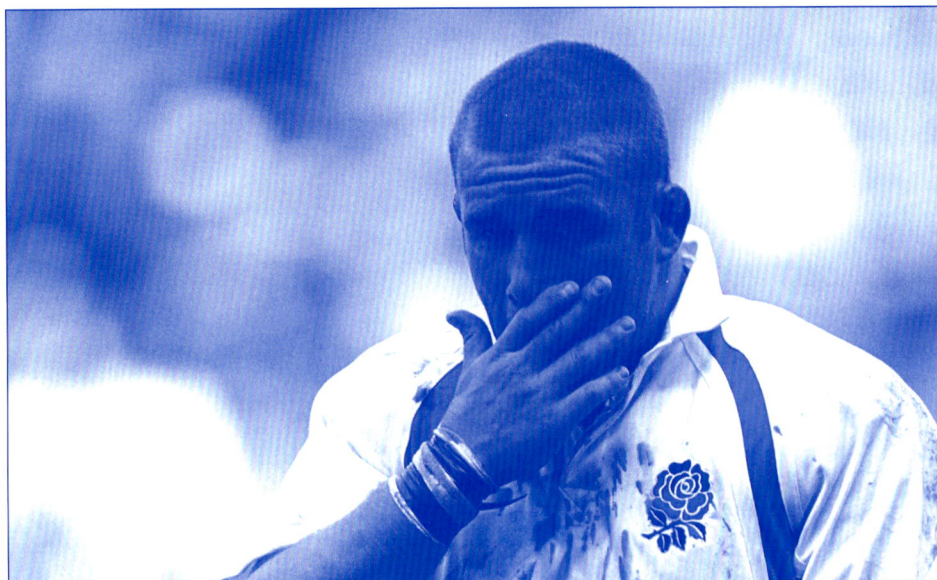

actionplus

EYE INJURIES

Eye injuries are common in sport, especially football, golf, squash and badminton. Inexperienced players and children are particularly vulnerable. Use of protective wide vision eye guards should be encouraged in squash and badminton.

CHECKLIST FOR INITIAL ASSESSMENT

- Do the circumstances indicate injury or a foreign body (eg dirt or eyelash in the eye)?

- Is there blood in or around the eye?

- Is there impairment of vision?

▶▶ ACTION

- If the eye is injured, cover the closed eye with a clean dressing and remove casualty to hospital.

- A foreign body can be washed out with clean running water, or removed with a moistened swab or damp corner of a clean handkerchief.

- If a foreign body is under the upper eyelid, ask casualty to look down, grasp the upper lid by the lashes and draw it out and down over the lower lid. If the object is still there, bathe the eye and ask casualty to blink. If unsuccessful, take or send the casualty to hospital.

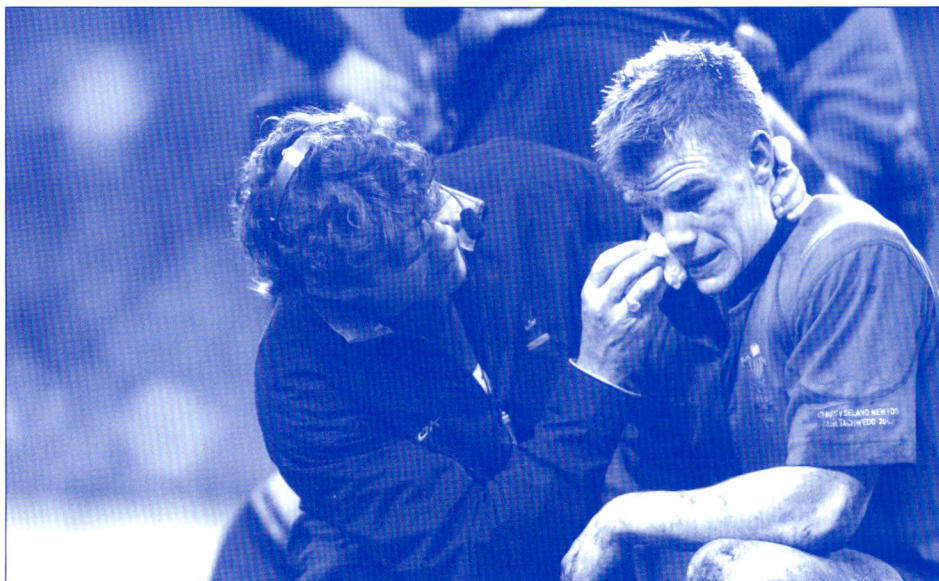

CHEST AND ABDOMINAL INJURIES

The chest and abdomen contain most of the body's vital organs. Injury to the chest may seriously interfere with breathing while damage to the abdomen may result in dangerous internal bleeding.

CHECKLIST FOR INITIAL ASSESSMENT

- Is the casualty able to breathe adequately?

- Is breathing painful?

- Look at colour of face and condition of skin. Is skin pale, cold, sweaty?

- Is there evidence of blood coughed up, or passed in urine?

- Observe pulse and breathing at intervals – increasing rates indicate loss of blood from the circulation.

- Look for bruising and tenderness.

- Check front of abdomen for rigidity.

IMPORTANT

Some of these factors may take several hours to develop. Therefore act on suspicion if the circumstances of the incident indicate possibility of internal injury.

▶▶ACTION

- If casualty has difficult and/or painful breathing, support in a half sitting position, turned onto the injured side (see Figure 10). Do not give anything to eat or drink.

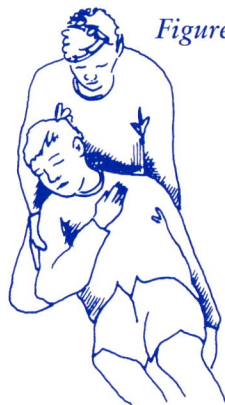

Figure 10

- Loosen clothing, particularly round the waist.

- If the casualty is pale and is breathing adequately, treat for shock. Arrange removal to hospital.

- Record pulse periodically and send this record with casualty to hospital.

- Monitor consciousness. If the casualty becomes unconscious, open the airway and check breathing for up to ten seconds. If the casualty is breathing, place in the recovery position onto the injured side. Be ready to resuscitate if necessary.

WINDING

A blow in the pit of the stomach or having the chest crushed can cause a participant to become winded. Participants find they cannot breathe in and lie gasping for breath. It is important not to interfere with participants in these circumstances. Allow them to recover their own breath, which usually takes approximately one minute, constantly reassuring them. Loosen any tight clothing and lightly massage the abdomen of the injured participant.

INJURIES TO THE FEMALE BREAST

The breast can be damaged in either running or contact sports. It is important to ensure that women participating in sport, wear an appropriate form of protective and supportive bra which does not damage the nipples.

Any bruise of the breast will always tend to settle in the lower half of the breast and may form a breast lump. It is important that any breast lump should be examined by a doctor, irrespective of whether or not you may relate it to an injury.

SPINAL INJURY

The spine is made up of a column of bones called vertebrae, which are separated by discs which act as shock absorbers. The spinal column is held together by ligaments and is supported by the muscles of the trunk.

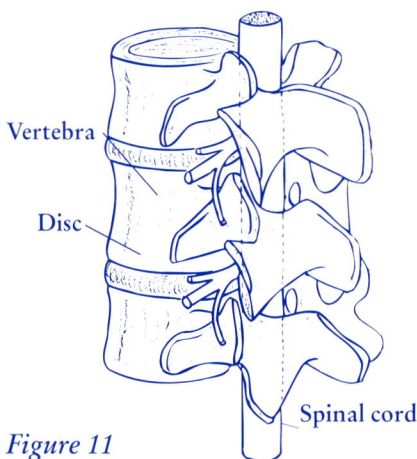

Vertebra

Disc

Spinal cord

Figure 11

The spinal cord extends from the brain and passes through a canal formed by the vertebrae (Figure 11). It is a very delicate structure and if damaged can result in loss or disturbance of power or sensation in some or all parts of the body below the injured area. This may be temporary but will be permanent if the cord is partially or completely severed.

Therefore the greatest care must be taken in dealing with a neck or back injury when fracture is suspected.

The two most vulnerable areas of the spinal column are the neck and lower back. In sport the most common activities in which spinal injuries occur are diving, rugby, football, gymnastics, trampolining, horse riding and motor sport.

CHECKLIST FOR INITIAL ASSESSMENT

- Do circumstances of the accident suggest possibility of spinal injury? Even apparently simple falls can result in severe damage.

- Establish site and severity of pain.

- Ask casualty to move wrists/ankles, fingers/toes gently. Movement may be weak.

- Establish if any tenderness around the back.

- Test sensation by gently touching limbs below site of injury.

- Ask if tingling/numb sensation or shooting pains are felt.

REMEMBER

Spinal injury is not excluded by absence of the above signs. Any disturbance of feeling or movement (however slight or however temporary) should raise the possibility of a spinal fracture or spinal cord injury.

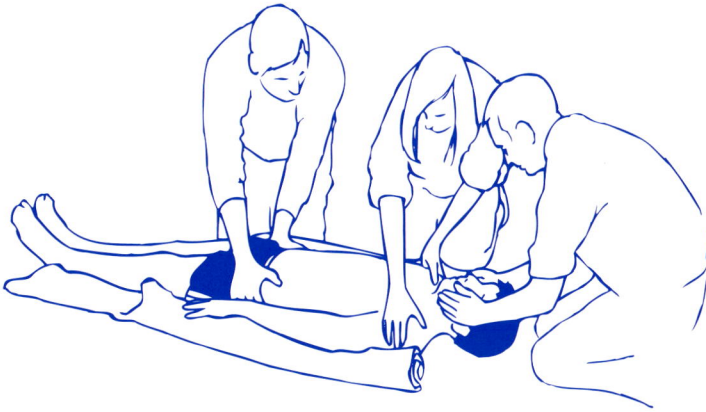

Figure 12

▶▶ ACTION

- **Do not move casualty unless their life is in danger. Wait for expert help to arrive. If movement of the casualty is imperative, use plenty of helpers to ensure the spine is moved in one piece and kept in alignment.**

- **Reassure casualty and tell not to move.**

- **Maintain position in which found unless danger or priority of airway, breathing or circulation dictate otherwise.**

- **Call an ambulance.**

- Steady and support head and neck in neutral position by placing your hands over casualty's ears. Get bystanders to support shoulders and hips (Figure 12).

- Clothing or rolled blankets alongside will give added support.

- Cover with blanket to minimise shock and keep warm.

- Support of head and neck must be maintained by hands until arrival at hospital.

If the casualty is unconscious and spinal injury suspected:

- Check breathing for up to ten seconds. If casualty not breathing, open airway by jaw lift (minimising movement of neck). If this is unsuccessful, tilt head slightly.

- Carry out resuscitation procedures as necessary.

- If breathing, place in recovery position with great care, minimising movement of neck (see page 22).

SHOULDER AND UPPER LIMB

The shoulder girdle and upper limbs consist of the shoulder blade (scapula), the collar bone (clavicle), the upper arm (humerus), forearm (radius and ulna), the wrist and the hand. They are covered with powerful muscles.

There are two joints in the region of the shoulder, the shoulder joint itself and the small joint between the collar bone and the shoulder blade (acromioclavicular) which lies on top of the shoulder joint.

The stability of the shoulder joint depends on the cuff of muscles attached to the top of the humerus (the rotator cuff). The muscles and tendons around the shoulder joint are commonly strained and should receive basic soft tissue injury treatment. Medical advice may also be required.

FRACTURE OF THE COLLAR BONE (CLAVICLE)

This usually results from a fall on to the point of the shoulder, or more rarely, the elbow or outstretched hand. It is the most common of all fractures and occurs at all ages.

CHECKLIST FOR INITIAL ASSESSMENT

- Checklist as for bone and joint injuries (see page 40).
- Does casualty support the arm of injured side with head inclined towards it?
- Is casualty reluctant to move the arm of injured side?
- Is there swelling or deformity at site of injury?

▶▶ ACTION

- Support and immobilise the upper limb (see page 70–71).
- Remove casualty to hospital.

ACROMIO-CLAVICULAR JOINT INJURY

This joint is usually injured by a fall on to the top of the shoulder. It may simply be sprained with pain and little or no swelling, or be subluxed (partially dislocated) or dislocated with a visible swelling or step-like deformity. This injury is common in young adults, especially in rugby and wrestling.

CHECKLIST FOR INITIAL ASSESSMENT

- Checklist as for bone and joint injuries (see page 40).
- Is there deformity as described above?

▶▶ ACTION

- Support and immobilise the upper limb (see page 70–71).
- Apply an ice pack or cold pad.
- Remove casualty to hospital.

FOLLOW-UP ADVICE

Following a sprain, if pain increases or progress is slow, seek medical advice.

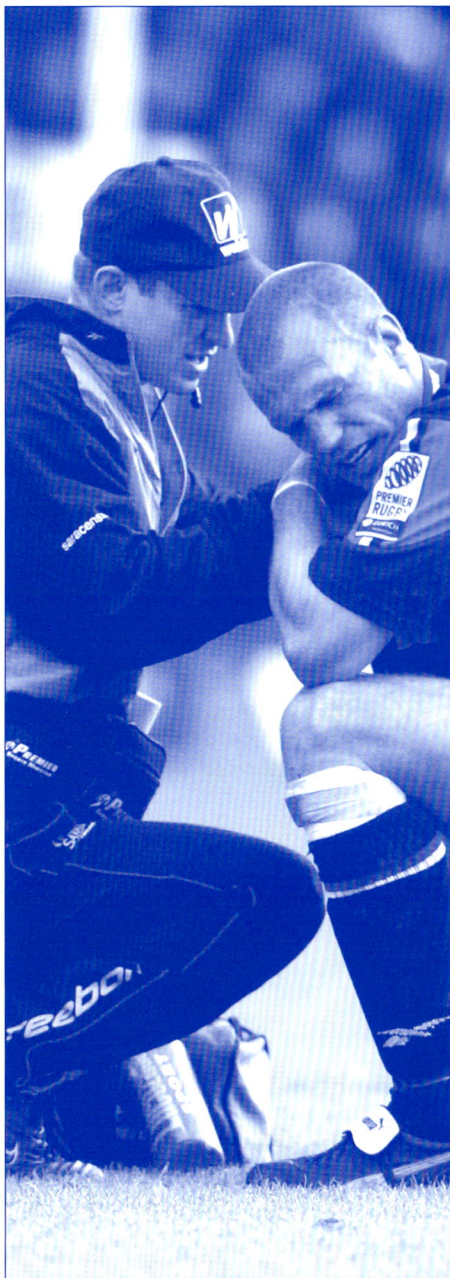

actionplus

DISLOCATED SHOULDER

A dislocation of the shoulder joint is caused by a fall on the outstretched hand, elbow or the point of the shoulder. Typically the shoulder will lose its normal round appearance and take on a more square shape (Figure 13).

Figure 13

(1) Undamaged Shoulder

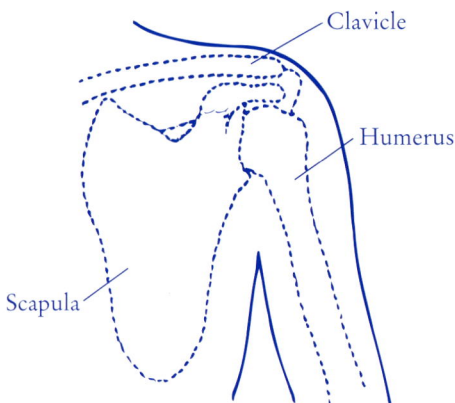

(2) Damaged Shoulder

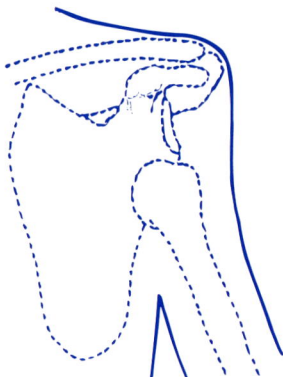

In a few instances, dislocation may be associated with damage to nerves, giving tingling or numbness in the arm and hand.

Some patients suffer with recurrent dislocation of the shoulder. In such cases the joint can dislocate with relatively little force. Most of these eventually need surgery which leaves them with a slight restriction of movement.

CHECKLIST FOR INITIAL ASSESSMENT

- Is the typical deformity present?

▶▶ACTION

- Support the arm in an arm sling.
- Remove the casualty to hospital without delay.

FRACTURE OF THE UPPER ARM BONE (HUMERUS)

This fracture results from a direct blow, a fall on to the arm or from the arm being twisted or bent.

CHECKLIST FOR INITIAL ASSESSMENT

- Checklist as for bone and joint injuries (see page 40).

▶▶ ACTION

- Support and immobilise the injured limb (see page 70–71).
- Remove casualty to hospital.

DISLOCATION OF THE ELBOW

This injury is caused by falling on to the outstretched hand. The forearm is driven backwards on the upper arm, making the tip of the elbow more prominent. This may also produce nerve injury with tingling or numbness in the fingers and hand, or interference with circulation to the hand.

CHECKLIST FOR INITIAL ASSESSMENT

- Is the above deformity present?
- Is the pulse present at the wrist?

▶▶ ACTION

- Support the arm comfortably. Use an arm sling if the elbow is bent.
- Remove the casualty to hospital without delay.

TENNIS AND GOLFER'S ELBOW

Pain on the outside of the elbow occurs in the condition known as tennis elbow. It is an overuse injury which is not only produced in racket sports but can occur with any repetitive movement. It is best treated by rest for a few days, ice packs, mild pain-relieving tablets and supporting strapping to the muscles of the forearm.

If the symptoms do not settle in a few days, seek medical advice. Try to identify the cause of the problem such as an inappropriate technique or equipment.

Golfer's elbow affects the inside of the elbow and the cause and treatment are similar to tennis elbow.

FRACTURE OF THE FOREARM AND WRIST

This is caused in a similar manner to fractures of the humerus.

CHECKLIST FOR INITIAL ASSESSMENT

• Checklist as for the bone and joint injuries (see page 40).

▶▶ ACTION

• Support and immobilise the injured part (see page 70–71).

• Remove the casualty to hospital.

SPRAINS OF THE THUMB

The ligaments at the base of the thumb are frequently injured in sport when the thumb is caught and twisted or bent. If completely torn these ligaments usually require surgical repair. A complete tear should be suspected if there is severe swelling or if bruising appears.

CHECKLIST FOR INITIAL ASSESSMENT

- Is the swelling severe?
- Is there any bruising?
- Is the pain severe?

▶▶ACTION

- If the answers are *no*, then treat as ligament sprain (see page 38).
- If the answer to any of these questions is *yes*, apply a supporting bandage and an elevation sling and remove the casualty to hospital.

SPRAINS OF THE FINGER JOINTS

These joints are frequently injured in sports, particularly those involving hand contact. If the joint moves abnormally (from side to side), the ligament is completely torn.

CHECKLIST FOR INITIAL ASSESSMENT

- Is there abnormal movement?

▶▶ACTION

- If the answer is *yes*, remove the casualty to hospital.
- If the answer is *no*, tape lightly to adjoining fingers while still allowing movement of the finger joint. If swelling persists, advise casualty to speak to a doctor.

FOLLOW-UP ADVICE

Spindle shaped swelling and discomfort may persist for several months. In these circumstances, advise casualty to seek medical advice and to protect the injured finger by strapping to adjoining finger when participating in sport over the next few months.

DISLOCATION OF THE FINGERS

If twisting or bending force is severe, dislocation of finger joints may occur. There is an obvious step-shaped deformity of the affected joint.

CHECKLIST FOR INITIAL ASSESSMENT

• Is deformity present?

▶▶ACTION

• A firm steady pull on the displaced part along the line of the finger usually allows the dislocation to slip back into place. This may be attempted once. If successful, assess and treat as for sprains of the finger. If unsuccessful, remove casualty to hospital.

MALLET FINGER

A sharp blow on the top of the finger while it is straight (eg from a ball), may force forward the joint at the end of the finger. This can damage or tear the tendon which holds the finger straight and this joint drops.

CHECKLIST FOR INITIAL ASSESSMENT

• Is deformity present?
• Is the casualty unable to straighten the finger tip?

▶▶ACTION

• Seek medical advice.

PELVIC GIRDLE AND LOWER LIMB INJURIES

Each lower limb consists of the thigh bone (femur), the leg bones (tibia and fibula) and the bones at the ankle and foot. The kneecap (patella) is a bone which lies within the large tendon on the front of the knee which straightens the knee.

The femur is joined to the pelvic girdle at the hip joint which is a very stable ball and socket joint and covered by many muscles.

The knee joint is a shallow joint, deepened on each side by a cartilage (meniscus) and entirely supported by ligaments and tendons.

The ankle joint is supported on each side by ligaments and tendons. Many bones make up the arch of the foot. They are small and entirely supported by ligaments and tendons. For this reason the foot requires to be supported in good quality footwear appropriate to the sporting activity.

DISLOCATION OF THE HIP

This is an uncommon injury in sport but may occur if the leg is driven backwards on the pelvis. There is usually extreme pain in the hip and the leg characteristically lies bent forwards at the hip, turned inwards and tending to lie over the other leg.

CHECKLIST FOR INITIAL ASSESSMENT

- Is the characteristic deformity present?

▶▶ACTION

- Do not attempt to straighten or splint the leg.

- Support the limb comfortably in the position found.

- Arrange removal to hospital without delay.

TESTICULAR INJURIES

The testicles are suspended in a vulnerable position. A blow in the testicles is sickeningly painful. Usually the pain passes quite quickly, but if pain persists a doctor should be consulted as soon as possible. If a participant develops pain in a testicle while training or playing without sustaining an injury, he should see a doctor as soon as possible.

GROIN STRAIN

Groin strain is a complex problem arising in sport and has many different causes. It usually involves inflammation or strain of the tendons of the thigh or abdomen where they are attached to the bones of the pelvis or the femur.

Groin strain is a chronic problem, best treated by rest with advice from a chartered physiotherapist or doctor. The cause of the condition must be identified and eliminated from the affected person's exercise pattern.

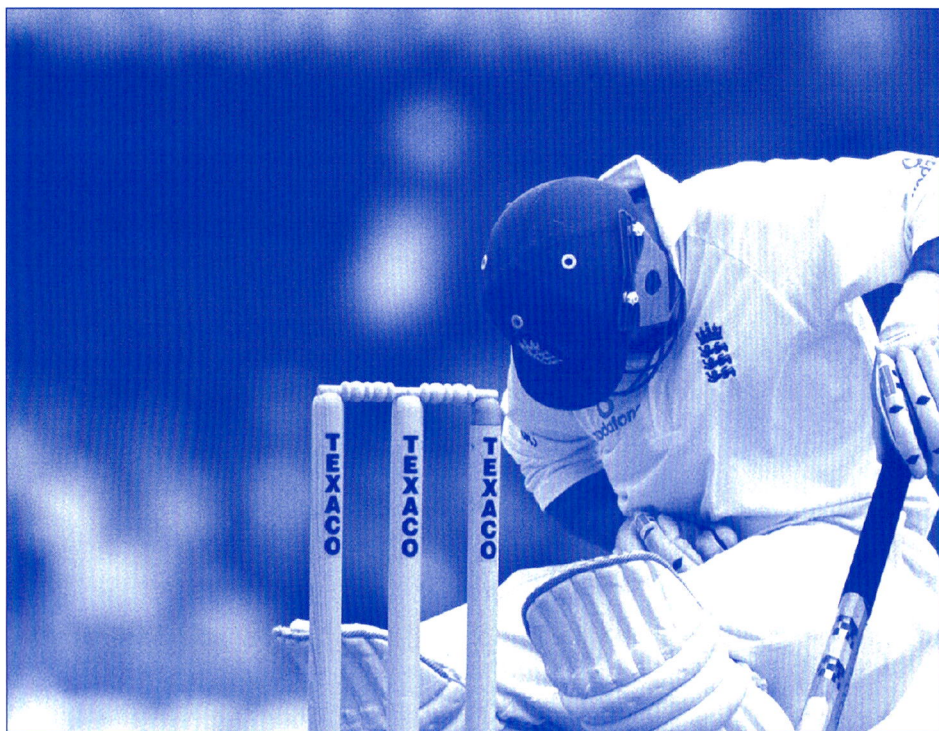

actionplus

PELVIC FRACTURE

These fractures can result from crushing or indirect force.

CHECKLIST FOR INITIAL ASSESSMENT

- Checklist as for bone and joint injuries (see page 40)
- Is the casualty unable to walk although legs appear sound?
- Blood at the urinary orifice, inability to pass urine or painful to do so?

▶▶ ACTION

- Help the casualty to lie on their back with legs straight or slightly bent and supported if more comfortable
- Immobilise the legs by bandaging them together and padding any bony points
- Arrange removal to hospital without delay.

FRACTURE OF THE THIGH OR LEG

These fractures result from a violent injury.

CHECKLIST FOR INITIAL ASSESSMENT

- Checklist as for bone and joint injuries (see page 40).

▶▶ ACTION

- Handle the limb gently with adequate support.
- Loosely cover any wound with a suitable, sterile dressing.
- Immobilise the injured limb (see page 73).
- Arrange removal to hospital without delay.

INJURIES OF THE KNEE

PAIN IN THE KNEECAP

Also known as *anterior knee pain*, *patello-femoral pain* and *chondromalacia patellae*.

The condition results from abnormal rubbing of the back of the kneecap on the lower end of the thighbone (femur) due to a combination of factors including imbalanced pull of the muscles at the front of the knee. It is most common in runners and jumpers, especially in women, which may be due to certain anatomical differences in the shape of their pelvis.

Pain is experienced behind the kneecap and often associated with a creaking noise which occurs during or after exercise, or going up and down stairs. The acute pain can be relieved by the application of an ice pack and taking mild pain-relieving tablets. However, prevention requires a carefully balanced muscle training programme to build up the muscle on the inner aspect at the front of the lower thigh. This is best supervised by a chartered physiotherapist.

Figure 14

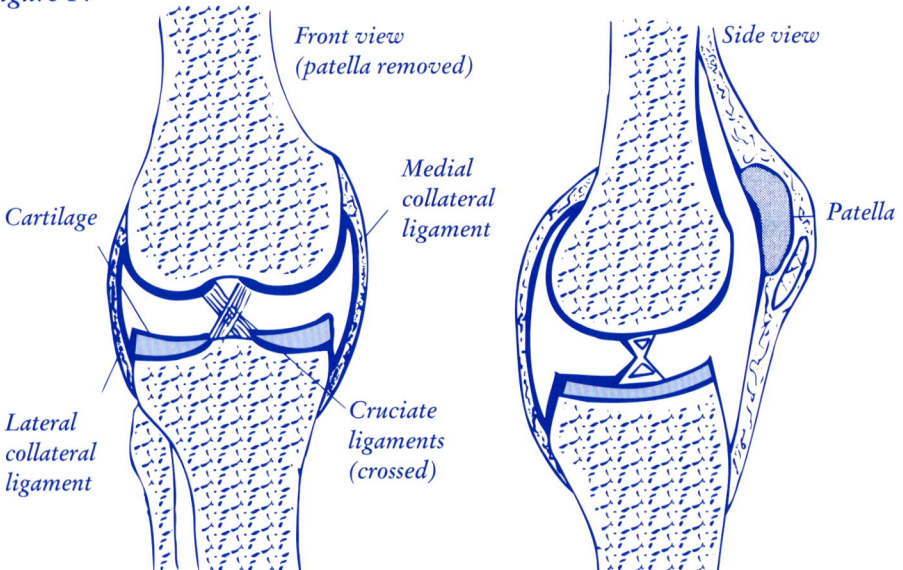

Front view (patella removed)

Side view

Cartilage

Medial collateral ligament

Patella

Lateral collateral ligament

Cruciate ligaments (crossed)

KNEE PAIN IN CHILDREN

In addition to any of the preceding conditions, children can develop pain and swelling localised to the normal prominence on the front of the upper shin just below the kneecap during and after activity. It is due to the large tendon at the front of the knee pulling on the growing part of the bone. It will settle completely once the child is fully grown, but during the painful period symptoms can be controlled by reduction in exercise.

CHECKLIST FOR INITIAL ASSESSMENT

- Pain over the upper shin on activity?
- Is there swelling and tenderness where the tendon joins the upper shin?

▶▶ACTION

- Reduce activities.
- If the symptoms are severe or do not settle, seek medical advice.
- Increasing pain and swelling in a child's knee should always be investigated by a specialist.

LIGAMENT INJURIES

There is a large ligament on each side of the knee (collateral ligaments) and two within the knee joint (cruciate ligaments) (Figure 14).

The collateral ligaments (on either side) are injured by any force which pushes or twists the knee in an abnormal direction.

This injury may be a simple sprain which requires treatment by the basic principles used to treat soft tissue injuries (see page 36). A more severe force will rupture the ligament completely and allow abnormal side to side movement at the knee. It most commonly affects the inner (medial) ligament and requires hospital treatment. Cruciate ligament injuries occur as a complication of the severe collateral ligament injury described above, or following a direct blow to the front of the shin or knee. A cruciate ligament injury requires hospital treatment.

CHECKLIST FOR INITIAL ASSESSMENT

- How did the injury occur?
- Is there obvious swelling in the knee joint soon after the injury?
- Is there abnormal side to side, or back and forward movement?

▶▶ ACTION

- If either abnormality is present, support the knee in the most comfortable position and remove the casualty to hospital without delay.

TORN CARTILAGE (MENISCUS)

There are two half moon shaped cartilages in the knee, one on either side, which act as shock absorbers. They may be torn if the leg is violently twisted at the knee while bearing weight. This may cause the knee to lock or give way. It is an extremely common injury in football and may be associated with damage to the corresponding collateral ligament as described above.

CHECKLIST FOR INITIAL ASSESSMENT

- How did the injury occur?
- Is complete straightening or bending of the knee restricted?
- Is the pain and tenderness mainly on one side of the knee?

▶▶ ACTION

- If either abnormality is present, apply supporting strapping and seek medical advice.

Note: A good guide as to the severity of a joint injury is how quickly the joint swells after the injury. A rapid development of swelling (within 10–30 minutes) may be due to bleeding in the cavity of the joint and is called a haemarthrosis. Slow development of swelling (over several hours) is due to an accumulation of synovial fluid from the synovial membrane, and is known as a synovial effusion. Bleeding in the joint is a severe injury and should be referred directly to hospital.

SHIN SPLINTS

Many middle distance runners experience pain in the front of the leg which is known as shin splints. The pain can be due to several different causes including inflammation of the muscles and tendons attached to the shin, or to stress fracture of the leg bone (tibia or fibula). Any athlete presenting with soft tissue shin splints should reduce the training programme, run on a soft surface (eg grass) and check the quality of shoes is appropriate to the workload undertaken. However, stress fractures need at least four and probably eight to twelve weeks to heal. They are likely to be aggravated by continued running, although walking should do no harm.

If these measures do not ease the symptoms, seek appropriate medical advice.

ACUTE COMPARTMENT SYNDROME

Occasionally sportspeople can complain of lower leg pain associated with a feeling of numbness and weakness in the foot. This is due to swelling of the muscles impairing circulation. It may manifest as a form of **shin splints**.

CHECKLIST FOR INITIAL ASSESSMENT

• Is the pain increased by movement of the toes or foot?

• Does the pain last for a few minutes after stopping the activity which caused it?

▶▶ ACTION

• Make an appointment to see the doctor in case it is necessary to see a consultant specialising in sports medicine. If the pain is severe and acute compartment syndrome is suspected, the patient should be taken directly to hospital.

ACHILLES TENDON INJURIES

The achilles tendon joins the calf muscles to the heel and works vigorously, lifting the body weight upwards and forwards during walking or running. The tendon may rupture during activity and this is often described as feeling like a kick on the back of the ankle.

A more common and very complex problem, especially in runners, is inflammation and degeneration in the tendon itself (tendinitis), or the fine sheath around the tendon (paratendinitis) which is aggravated by exercise.

ACHILLES TENDINITIS

CHECKLIST FOR INITIAL ASSESSMENT

- Is there swelling of the tendon?
- Is there tenderness of the tendon?

▶▶ ACTION

- If acute, treat as tendon injury (see page 63).
- If chronic, reduce activity and run on soft surfaces; check on sports footwear.
- If no improvement, seek medical advice.

RUPTURE OF THE ACHILLES TENDON

CHECKLIST FOR INITIAL ASSESSMENT

- How did the injury occur?
- Is there a gap which can be felt in the tendon?
- Can the toe and the foot be actively pointed downwards?

▶▶ ACTION

- If suspicious, remove casualty to hospital.

ANKLE INJURIES

Twisting injuries of the ankle are common in all sports and frequently result in damage to the ligaments on either side of the ankle (usually the outside).

Most injuries, particularly those affecting the outside of the joint, are sprains (Figure 15).

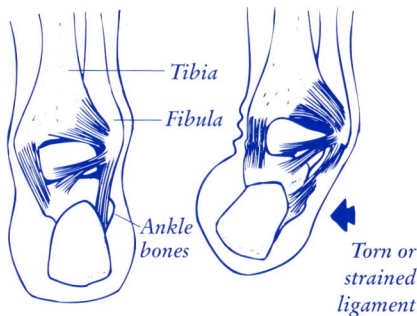

Figure 15

A severe twisting injury of the ankle can result in fracture of the bones.

CHECKLIST FOR INITIAL ASSESSMENT

- Is the casualty unable to walk?
- Is there a great deal of swelling?
- Are there signs to suggest a fracture?

▶▶ ACTION

- If the answer to any of the above is *yes*, immobilise the limb (see page 73) and seek medical advice.
- If the answer to all the above is *no*, treat as a minor sprain (see page 38).

Anyone with a minor sprain should be encouraged to walk in a normal fashion. It better to walk slowly with a normal heel to toe gait, putting the ankle through as full a range of movement as possible. This will reduce strain injuries higher in the leg.

FOLLOW-UP ADVICE

During recovery, attention should be paid to exercises which strengthen the leg muscles, restore full range of movement and improve balance and coordination. This will minimise the limp and help to avoid recurrent injuries of the ankle.

FOOT PROBLEMS

Pain in the foot is frequently related to sprain of the ligaments supporting the bones which make up the arch of the foot. The pain is aggravated by inappropriate footwear with insufficient arch support.

Any sportsperson with foot problems should reduce the training programme, run on a soft surface (eg grass) and check that the footwear gives adequate arch support.

If the problem continues, suggest referral to a specialist.

Section Four

4

Practical
Procedures

SLINGS

ARM SLING

This sling is used to support the upper limb with the forearm slightly above horizontal, when the upper limb is injured or in some chest injuries.

- Sit the casualty down. Ask her to support the injured arm. Slide one end of the triangular bandage through the hollow under the elbow. Pull the upper end until it rests by the collar bone on the injured side (Figure 16).

Figure 16

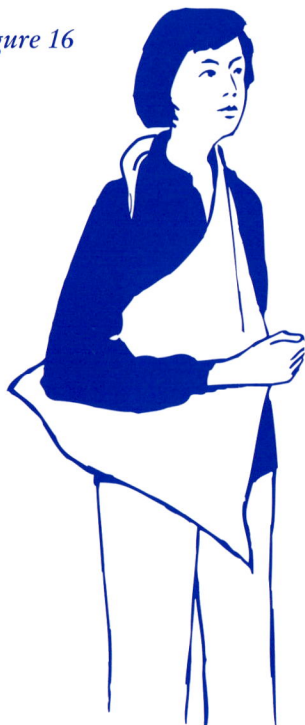

- Bring the lower end of the bandage up over the forearm so that the injured arm is now supported by the bandage.

- Tie a reef knot in the hollow above the collarbone on the injured side and then tuck the ends of the bandage under the reef knot.

- Tuck the excess bandage behind the elbow and secure the point with either a safety pin (Figure 17) or a twist.

Figure 17

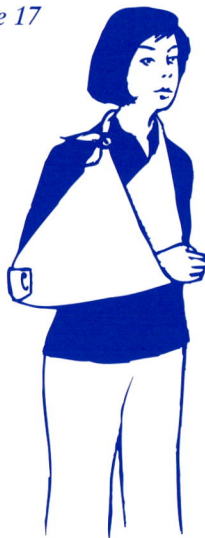

IMPORTANT

Always keep the casualty's injured arm well supported until the sling is secure and supports the arm itself.

ELEVATION SLING

This sling is used to support the upper limb with the hand at the opposite shoulder, when the hand is injured, or in some shoulder or chest injuries.

- Support the injured arm. Place the limb of the injured side on the chest with the fingertips at the opposite shoulder.

- Place an open triangular bandage over the limb with the point beyond the elbow and one end a short distance over the shoulder of the uninjured side (Figure 18).

- Tuck the base of the bandage under the hand and forearm.

- Carry the lower end across the back and tie the ends in a reef knot so that it lies in the hollow above the collarbone of the uninjured side (Figure 19).

- Tuck the point between the forearm and the front of the bandage; twist it or use a safety pin (Figure 20). Check the circulation in the thumb by pressing the skin until pale. If the colour does not return, loosen the bandage.

Figure 18

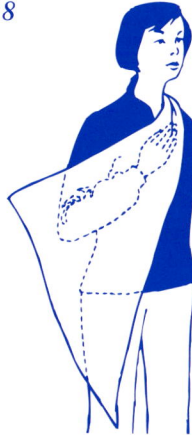

Figure 19

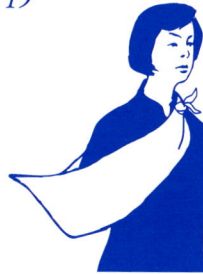

Figure 20

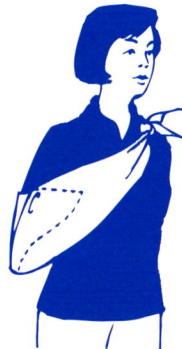

IMMOBILISATION OF LIMBS

UPPER LIMB

Fractures at the shoulder or in the hand:

- Sit the casualty down.
- If hand injured, control bleeding, put a dressing on and protect with soft padding.
- Support limb in elevation sling (see Page 69).
- Place soft padding between the limb and chest (Figure 21).

- Secure the limb to chest with broad-fold bandage applied over the sling (Figure 22).
- Check circulation and sensation in limb at 10 to 15 minute intervals.
- Take or send casualty to hospital.

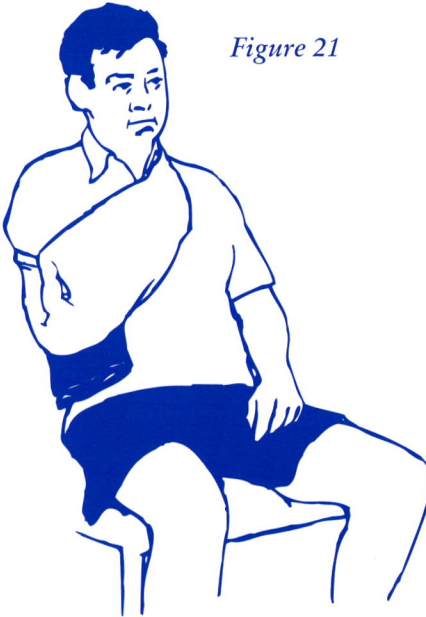

Figure 21

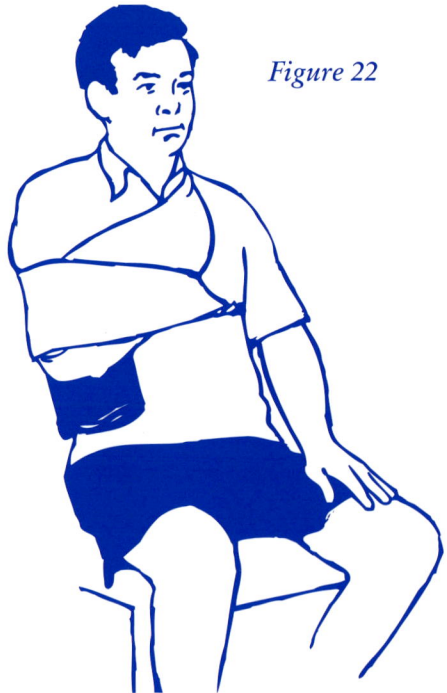

Figure 22

Fractures in arm or forearm:

- Seat the casualty comfortably. If possible, bend casualty's arm at elbow so that arm is across his trunk.

- Place soft padding between arm and chest. If forearm is injured, cradle it in soft padding (Figure 23).

Figure 23

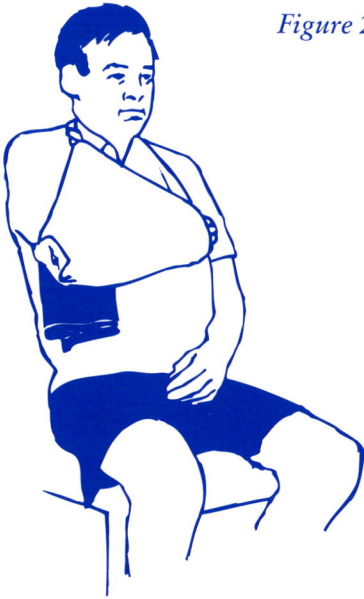

- Support the limb in arm sling (see page 68).

- Secure limb to chest with broad-fold bandage applied over sling avoiding fracture site (Figure 24).

Figure 24

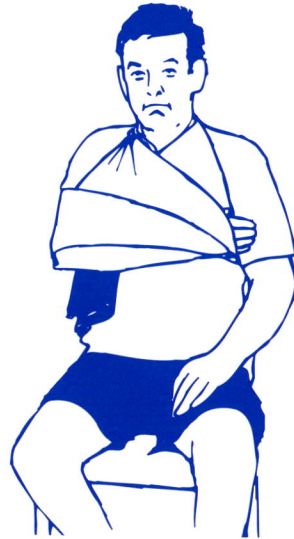

- Check circulation and sensation in limb at 10 to 15 minute intervals.

If elbow cannot be bent without increasing the pain, or the casualty is lying down:

- make casualty comfortable lying down and pad around the elbow

- support the injured limb against trunk.

- Place broad bandages:
  - under waist and slide upwards so it will be at the arm above the fracture site
  - under waist and slide downwards so that it will be round the forearm
  - under knees and slide upwards so it will be round the wrist and hand.
- Place sufficient soft padding between limb and trunk so that any space is filled.
- Tie bandage round wrist, hand and body.
- Tie bandage round arm and body.
- Tie bandage round forearm and body (Figure 25).

- Arrange transport by ambulance to hospital as a stretcher case.
- Check circulation and sensation in limb frequently.

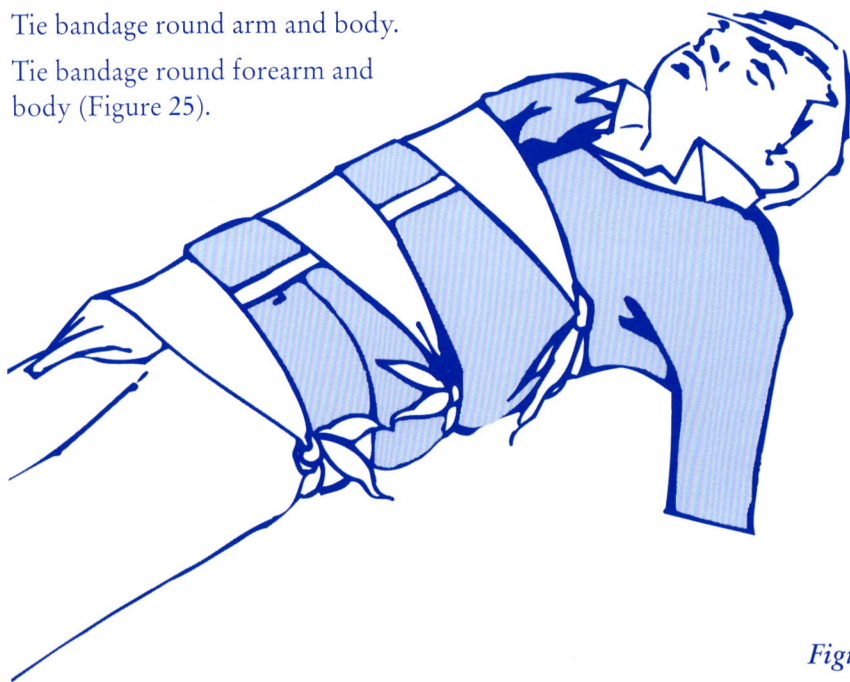

Figure 25

LOWER LIMB

If ambulance is expected quickly:

- steady and support limb by hand at joints above and below fracture site (Figure 26) or place cushions, rolled blanket or rug at side of limb to steady it.

Figure 26

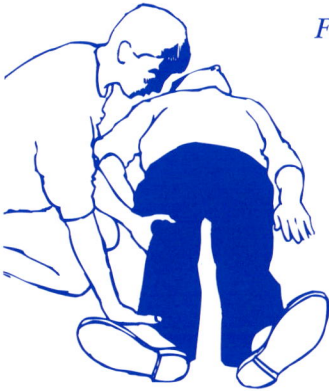

If arrival of ambulance will be delayed:

- continue support of limb; use four broad-fold bandages, place them under ankles and knees, above and below site of fracture (Figure 27).

Figure 27

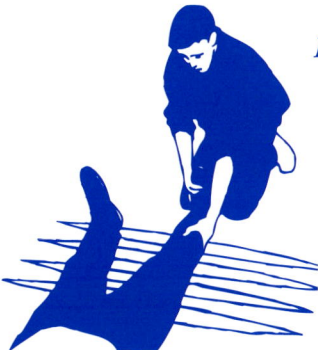

- Place adequate soft padding between limbs at knees and ankles and fill hollows between legs.

- Bring uninjured limb to side of injured limb.

- If it is necessary to adjust position of uninjured limb, apply gentle traction at foot before moving it.

- While support is maintained, apply bandage at ankles in figure eight round ankles and feet.

- Apply broad-fold bandage round knees, then above and below site of fracture. Tie knots on uninjured side (Figure 28).

If thigh bone is fractured, bandages are tied as above with the bandages above and below fracture site in thigh.

Check circulation and sensation in limb at 10–15 minute intervals.

Figure 28

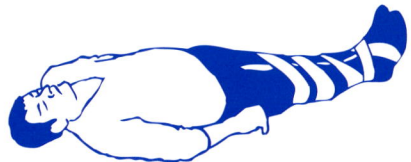

CERVICAL COLLAR

- While the casualty's head is being supported, fold newspaper to about 10 cms wide.

- Fold this paper round neck from the front so it supports the front and sides of the chin (Figure 29).

Figure 29

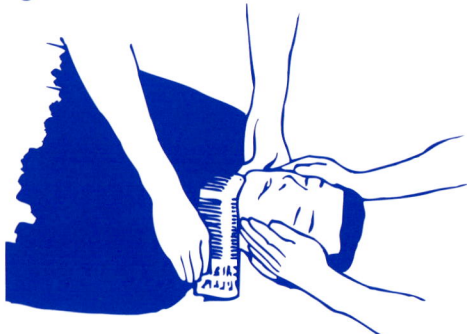

- Tie in place with neck tie or other means available (Figure 30).

- The initial manual support of the head should be continued until the ambulance arrives.

Figure 30

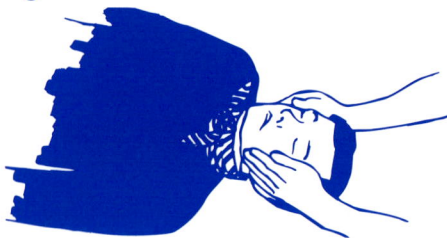

ICE

PURPOSE

Applying an ice pack or cold compress is useful in treating acute injuries. It will minimise the bleeding and swelling which occur in such injuries. It will also reduce pain.

METHOD OF APPLICATION

Always try to find out where you can get hold of an ice pack at your training or competition venue. Alternatively, you can buy special *instant ice packs* to keep in your first aid kit. If you do not have access to either of these, you can make a very effective cold compress as follows:

1 Fill a plastic bag half to two-thirds full of ice. Squeeze the air out of the plastic bag and then seal it (a bag of frozen peas or similar vegetable will also suffice).

2 Wrap the cold compress in a thin towel.

3 Place it over the casualty's injury and leave for about 30 minutes. The compress can either be left uncovered over the injury or secured in place with a compression bandage. Make sure the bandage does not become too tight and affect the circulation.

ADDITIONAL NOTES

The athlete must not return immediately to the sport as the apparent severity of the injury might be reduced by the pain-relieving effect of the ice.

To limit the damage:

* rest the injured part for 24–72 hours

* elevate whenever possible but especially at night

* support during the day with an elastic bandage.

To limit the damage follow the RICE procedure:

Rest

Ice

Compress

Elevate

* **Rest and raise the injury**

    Sit or lay the casualty down and rest the injured part in a comfortable position

* **Apply a cold compress to the affected limb**
    Apply an ice pack or cold pad to reduce blood flow and minimise swelling

* **Compress the injury with some soft padding**
    Apply gentle pressure by compressing the injury with soft padding or securing the compress with a bandage

* **Elevate the injured limb**
    Raise and support the casualty's injured limb to minimise any bruising. If the injury is to the casualty's wrist, elbow or shoulder, support the affected arm with an arm sling.

THE TRAINER'S MAGIC SPONGE

The magic sponge and bucket of water must never be used to clean damaged or infected skin. It is better to use sterile disposable swabs and dressings which can be discarded immediately after use.

Use once and discard safely.

PAIN-RELIEVING AEROSOLS

These products have only a superficial cooling effect and are expensive for what they achieve.

COMPRESSION BANDAGING

PURPOSE

The use of compression bandaging will inhibit swelling and, in doing so, may reduce the effect of an injury.

METHOD OF APPLICATION

The bandage should be as broad as possible (no less than 5cms in width). Place the injured part in a comfortable position. If available, a roll of cotton wool should be wrapped around the part and then the bandage applied over the cotton wool, starting away from the trunk and working towards it. The bandage should be firm enough to prevent movement and maintain even pressure over the part. It should not, however, restrict the circulation nor cause the patient any pain. If available, a crepe bandage or elastic consistency strapping should be used.

ADDITIONAL NOTES

The compression bandage should be removed at least every hour for five to ten minutes to allow the circulation to be maintained. It must be removed before sleeping.

ADHESIVE STRAPPING

Strapping should only be applied by those trained in its use.

PURPOSE

Adhesive strapping is used to limit joint movements which cause pain. It should not be used to allow activity which would otherwise be inadvisable and could aggravate an underlying injury.

METHOD OF APPLICATION

IMPORTANT – Enquiry should always be made about possible allergy to adhesive materials and the limb shaved before applying tape. Alternatively, the skin and hair can be protected by a single layer of bandage or under wrap.

Depending on the area, different widths and materials are used (eg on the thigh, 5.0 to 7.5cms wide elastic consistency strapping should be used, whereas for the ankle 2.5cms non-elastic consistency strapping is better). As a general rule, strapping should not be wound round the part but longitudinal strands placed on either side of the joint.

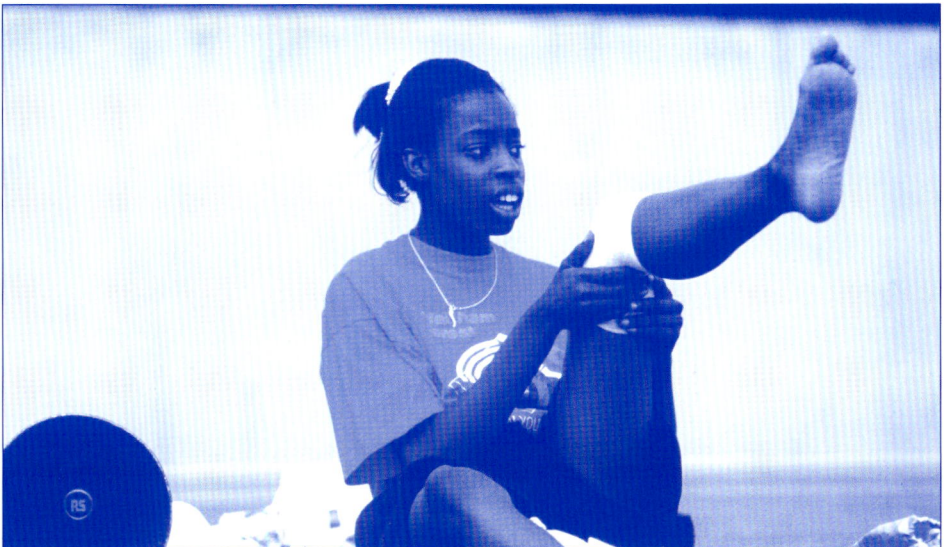

actionplus

HANDLING AND TRANSPORT

In sporting injuries a casualty will often be outdoors in inclement conditions. The casualty must be protected from the weather. After carrying out initial first aid procedures, in the absence of contraindications (eg spinal injury), the casualty should be moved to shelter (by stretcher if appropriate).

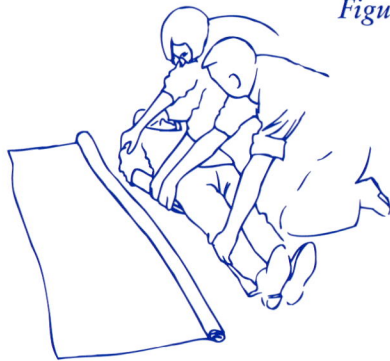

Figure 31

PLACING BLANKET UNDER CASUALTY

- Fold blanket to suitable thickness, bearing in mind that when lying on damp ground more insulation is required below than above.

- Roll folded blanket from side to centre.

- Place rolled edge of blanket close to casualty's side; the injured side if injuries are on one side. Kneel, with assistants if available, at other side of casualty (Figure 31).

- Gently turn casualty on to his side away from the blanket and support him on his side (Figure 32).

- Lift blanket to casualty, placing rolled edge close to casualty's back.

- Gently turn casualty on to his back on the blanket. Tilt casualty sufficiently to opposite side to allow the blanket to be unrolled from under him (Figure 33).

- Settle casualty comfortably on the blanket.

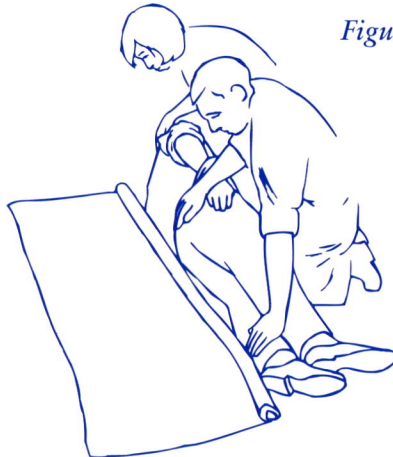

Figure 32

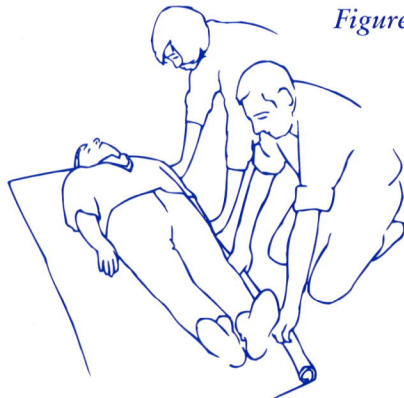

Figure 33

LOADING A STRETCHER USING FOUR PEOPLE

Before using a stretcher it should be tested by lifting an uninjured person of at least the same weight as the casualty.

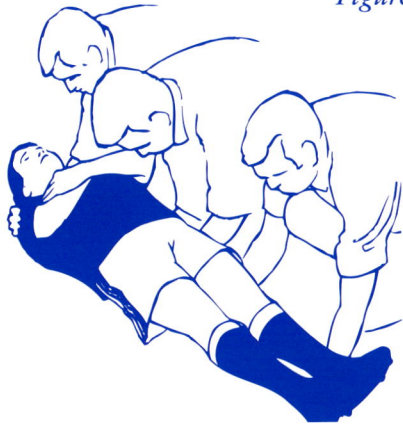

Figure 34

- The opened stretcher should be placed in line with the casualty's head. Three people should kneel on their left facing the casualty's left side at shoulders, hips and knees.

- Forearms should be placed under the casualty. The person at the top supports the head and shoulders, the middle person supports the small of the back and hips and the third person supports the thighs and legs (Figure 34).

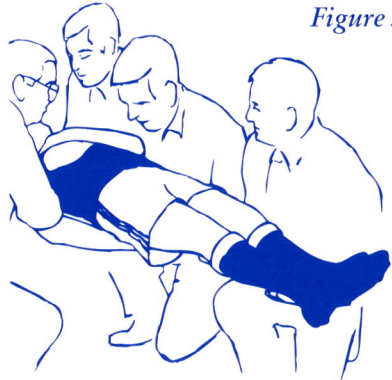

Figure 35

- The first aider in charge should kneel on the casualty's right side facing the chest, and provide additional support to the shoulders and trunk by grasping the wrists of the person opposite.

- When the first aider in charge gives the order to lift, the casualty should be raised slowly and evenly on to the right knees of the three people on the left (Figure 35). The stretcher is now placed below the casualty by a bystander or the first aider in charge.

Figure 36

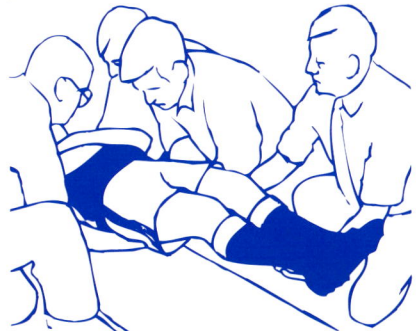

- On the order to lower, the casualty should be gently and evenly lowered on to the stretcher by all four people (Figure 36).

CARRYING A STRETCHER

A stretcher is best carried by four people (except through narrow doorways) with the casualty's feet forward and the person in charge at the front right handle.

- The bearers should stand close to the stretcher, grasping the handles with their inner hands and keeping their arms straight. The stretcher must be kept level while being lifted, carried and lowered.

- The bearers should move together on command, stepping off with the foot nearest the stretcher and walking with a short flat-footed step to carry the casualty smoothly (Figure 37).

- In the absence of a stretcher, a conscious casualty with a relatively minor ankle or foot injury can be carried to shelter by a two handed seat (Figures 38 and 39).

Figure 37

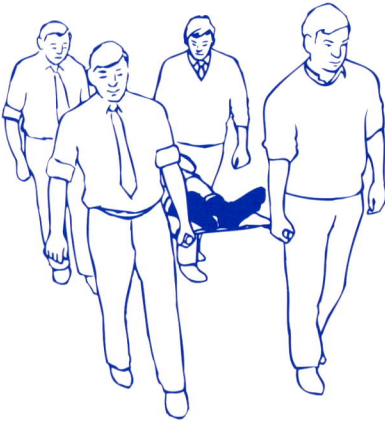

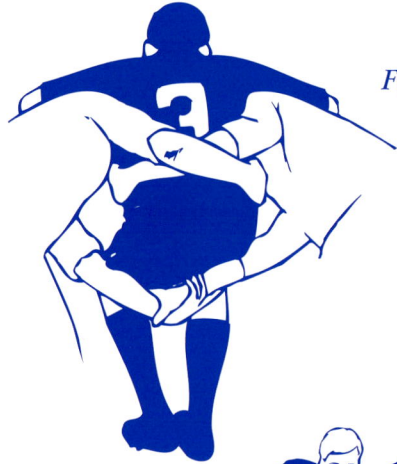

Figure 38

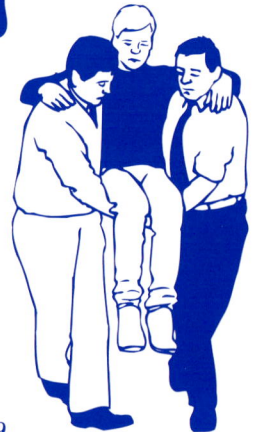

Figure 39

LOADING CASUALTY ON 'POLE AND CANVAS' STRETCHER

- Place the open stretcher alongside the casualty (on the injured side if injuries are on one side). Withdraw the pole nearer the casualty.

- Roll the canvas from the side nearest casualty to centre.

- Proceed as for placing blanket under casualty until casualty is lying on the stretcher canvas.

- Gently re-insert pole into sleeve of canvas.

REMEMBER!

Techniques for lifting and transporting casualties should not be used unless you have received comprehensive training from a qualified instructor.

If you have not, do not move the casualty unless his life is in danger – wait for expert help to arrive. Never risk your own safety to move a casualty.

LIFTING A CASUALTY FROM WATER (eg from a swimming pool or on to a boat)

If the casualty is suspected of having a neck or spinal injury, he should ideally be supported horizontally (eg on a board), floated to shallow water if possible, with head held in line with the trunk (see spinal injury page 48), then lifted out of the water horizontally with good support. If there is no reason to suspect a spinal injury, the casualty should be removed from the water without delay.

FIRST AID EQUIPMENT

All individuals participating in sport, as well as sports coaches, clubs and associations, should have their own first aid kit. The appropriate equipment will vary with the activity under consideration. An individual spending one hour a week jogging will require a minimum of equipment mainly designed to look after the feet, whereas a rugby or football club will require equipment for muscle, tendon and joint injuries as well as cuts and grazes.

Certain basic facilities and equipment should be available for all activities:

- Access to a telephone
- A supply of clean water

- Sealed sterile dressings
- Plasters
- Bandages
- Sterile gauze pads
- Adhesive tapes, safety pins, clips.

As well as the essential items, you may also wish to include a number of other items in your first aid kit:

- Tweezers
- Scissors
- Plastic disposable gloves
- Wound cleansing wipes
- Notepad and pencil
- Blanket.

It is important to repeat at this point that individuals, coaches and clubs have a responsibility to maintain the first aid equipment. There is nothing worse than having an injury to deal with and going to the first aid cupboard and finding it is bare.

Section Five

Returning to Sport

5

REHABILITATION

Injuries frequently recur, often as a result of incorrect advice or treatment, or because return to full activity was too soon. However, too prolonged a period of rest can be equally damaging. Recovery is an active process. The period of rehabilitation starts as soon as the injury has occurred, and the importance of correct immediate treatment has already been discussed. If medical advice has been sought, the doctor or physiotherapist will normally oversee the initial phase of rehabilitation and should be consulted before full training is resumed.

The first few days after an injury will involve a period of total rest of the injured part, but it is often possible to undertake some activity in order to maintain general fitness. For example, if you have a leg injury, you will normally be able to carry out an upper body exercise programme or non weight-bearing activity such as swimming.

A general fitness programme should be maintained while gradual progress is made to restore function in the injured part. For example, after a leg muscle injury, the following steps should be taken:

- Gentle muscle exercises, slowly increasing the range through which the muscle is used.
- Gentle stretching to the point of discomfort (not pain).
- Light weight training.
- Practising technical skills at a slow pace.
- Gradually increasing demands can then be made (eg striding, three-quarter pace sprinting, sprinting, changes of direction).
- Participation in full training should precede return to competition.

During the recovery programme it is important not to exercise beyond the point of pain.

It is better to take a little longer to return to full activity than to risk a recurrent or second and more serious injury, because of a lack of patience or trying to overcome a pain barrier. The programme is nearing completion when there is no longer pain, swelling or local heat; when full range of movement and full power of the muscle group has been restored.

Resting an injury too long, without efforts to restore normal function, can be equally damaging. Prolonged rest of active tissue results in loss of strength and poorly healed tissue.

The use of strapping is very controversial when an athlete is recovering from an injury. It can be used very successfully to support ligaments after a sprain. It should not be used to enable activities to be carried out which would otherwise cause pain. Generally, strapping should be used for a very limited period to support a joint.

All participants should be subjected to a fitness test before returning to vigorous or competitive activity. This type of functional test cannot be carried out in the medical room for it must simulate the type of pressures that will be incurred in the competitive/real situation. To devise such a test requires a comprehensive knowledge of the sport and a ruthless objectivity in assessing the performer's chances of completing the competition/activity without injury.

Sportspeople often lose confidence when they are injured. This is a particular problem in the case of recurring injuries.

It is vital that during the rehabilitation phase they continue to be involved with the sport as far as possible. They need plenty of support and encouragement (particularly from the coach) and, in the case of younger participants, from the parents.

Section Six

Where Next?

WHERE NEXT?

This resource and the accompanying **sports coach UK** Coach Workshop *Injury Prevention and Management* provide a general introduction to the steps which can be taken to avoid sports injuries and, when they arise, on how best to give immediate, safe treatment and care.

To continue to update and develop your knowledge, you are advised to take note of the workshops and resources recommended throughout the book. These will help to extend your knowledge further on specific topics. If you need further information on related subjects, you are recommended to refer to the following **sports coach UK** resources:

Workshop	Resource
The Body in Action (Introductory Workshop)	The Body in Action (Intro Study Pack)
Safety and Injury (Introductory Workshop)	Safety and Injury (Intro Study Pack)
Fuelling Performers (Coach Workshop)	Fuelling Performers (Handbook)
Fitness and Training (Coach Workshop)	Physiology and Performance (Handbook)
Emergency First Aid for Sport (in conjunction with British Red Cross)	Emergency First Aid for Sport (Handbook)
Field-based Fitness Testing (Performance Coach Workshop)	A Guide to Field Based Fitness Testing (Home Study Pack)
	Introduction to Sports Mechanics (Home Study Pack)
	Introduction to Sports Physiology (Home Study Pack)
	Introduction to the Structure of the Body (Home Study Pack)

All **sports coach UK** resources, along with 400 carefully selected sports-related products and resources are available from:

Coachwise 1st4sport
Chelsea Close
Off Amberley Road
Armley
Leeds
LS12 4HP

Tel: 0113-201 5555
Fax: 0113-231 9606

E-mail: enquiries@1st4sport.com Website: www.1st4sport.com

sports coach UK also produces a technical journal – *Faster, Higher, Stronger (FHS)* and an information update service for coaches – **sports coach update**. Details of these services are available from:

sports coach UK
114 Cardigan Road
Headingley
Leeds
LS6 3BJ

Tel: 0113-274 4802
Fax: 0113-275 5019

E-mail: coaching@sportscoachuk.org
Website: www.sportscoachuk.org

For details of all **sports coach UK** workshops, contact your nearest Regional Training Unit or home countries office. RTU contact details are available from **sports coach UK**.

For direct bookings on
sports coach UK workshops,
please contact:

scUK Workshop Booking Centre
Chelsea Close
Off Amberley Road
Armley
Leeds
LS12 4HP

Tel: 0845-601 3054
Fax: 0113-231 9606

AGENCIES AND ORGANISATIONS TO CONTACT

The purpose of this section is to identify a number of agencies and courses where coaches, parents and others can receive more detailed information on selected elements of this manual. The following are suggestions only and by no means represent an exhaustive list.

▶▶ National Sports Councils

sportscotland
Caledonia House
South Gyle
Edinburgh
EH12 9DQ

Tel: 0131-317 7200
Website: www.sportscotland.org.uk

UK Sport
40 Bernard Street
London
WC1N 1ST

Tel: 020-7211 5100
Website: www.uksport.gov.uk

Sport England
16 Upper Woburn Place
London
WCIH 0QP

Tel: 020-7273 1500
Website: www.sportengland.org

The Sports Council for Northern Ireland
House of Sport
Upper Malone Road
Belfast
BT9 5LA

Tel: 028-9038 1222
Website: www.sportni.org

Sports Council for Wales
The Welsh Institute of Sport
Sophia Gardens
Cardiff
CF11 9SW
Tel: 029-2030 0500
Website:
www.sports-council-wales.co.uk

▶▶ Voluntary First Aid Organisations

British Red Cross National Headquarters
9 Grosvenor Crescent
London
SW1X 7EJ

Tel: 020-7235 5454
Website: www.redcross.org.uk

St Andrew's Ambulance Association National Headquarters
48 Milton Street
Glasgow
G4 0HR

Tel: 0141-332 4031
Website: www.firstaid.org.uk

St John Ambulance National Headquarters
27 St John's Lane
London
EC1M 4BU

Tel: 020-7324 4000
Website: www.sja.org.uk

▶▶ National Outdoor Training Centres

sportscotland National Centre: Glenmore Lodge

Aviemore
Inverness-shire
PH22 1QU

Tel: 01479-861256
Website: www.glenmorelodge.org.uk

Plas y Brenin National Centre for Mountain Activities

Capel Curig
Conwy
North Wales
LL24 0ET

Tel: 01690-720214
Website: www.pyb.co.uk

Tollymore Mountain Centre

Bryansford
Newcastle
Co Down
BT33 0PT

Tel: 028-4372 2158
Website: www.tollymoremc.com

Plas Menai National Watersports Centre

Llanfairissgaer
Caernarfon
Gwynedd
LL55 1UE

Tel: 01248-670964
Website:
www.sports-council-wales.co.uk

sportscotland National Centre: Cumbrae

Isle of Cumbrae
Ayrshire
KA28 0HQ

Tel: 01475-530757
Website: www.sportscotland.org.uk

sportscotland National Centre: Inverclyde

Burnside Road
Largs
Ayrshire
KA30 8RW

Tel: 01475-674666
Website: www.sportscotland.org.uk

Holme Pierrepont National Water Sports Centre

Adbolton Lane
Holme Pierrepont
Nottingham
NG12 2LU

Tel: 0115-982 1212
Website:
www.leisureconnection.co.uk/holme

▶▶ Water Safety

Water Safety
Royal Life Saving Society UK
River House
High Street
Broom
Warwickshire
B50 4HN
Tel: 01789-773994
Website: www.rlss.org.uk

▶▶ Accident and Prevention

The Scottish Accident Prevention Council
Slateford House
53 Lanark Road
Edinburgh
EH14 1TL
Tel: 0131-455 7457
Website: www.sapc.org.uk

The Royal Society for the Prevention of Accidents (RoSPA)
Edgbaston Park
353 Bristol Road
Birmingham
B5 7ST
Tel: 0121-248 2000
Website: www.rospa.com

▶▶ Disability Organisations

British Paralympic Association

9th Floor
Norwich Union Building
69 Park Lane
Croydon
CR9 1BG

Tel: 020-7662 8882
Website: www.paralympics.org.uk

Disability Sport England

Unit 4E, N17 Studios
784 – 788 High Road
Tottenham
London
N1 6DX

Tel: 020-8801 4466
Website: www.disabilitysport.org.uk

English Sports Association for People with Learning Disabilities

Unit 9
Milner Way
Ossett
West Yorkshire
WF5 9JN

Tel: 01924-267 555
Website: www.esapld.co.uk

Scottish Disability Sport

Fife Sports Institute
Viewfield Road
Glenrothes
KY6 2RB

Tel: 01592-415700
Website: www.disabilitysport.com

Federation of Sports Association for the Disabled (Wales)

Welsh Institute of Sport
Sophia Gardens
Cardiff
CF11 9SW

Tel: 029-2030 0525/6
Website:
www.sports-council-wales.co.uk

Disability Sports Northern Ireland

Ormeau Business Park
8 Cromac Avenue
Belfast
BT7 2JA

Tel: 028-9050 8255
Website: www.dsni.co.uk

▶▶ Health Education

Health Development Agency
Holborn Gate
330 High Holborn
London
WC1V 7BA

Tel: 020-7430 0850
Website: www.hda-online.org.uk

The Health Education Board for Scotland
Woodburn House
Canaan Lane
Edinburgh
EH10 4SG

Tel: 0131-536 5500
Website: www.hebs.scot.nhs.uk

FURTHER PUBLICATIONS

▶▶ BRITISH RED CROSS ST ANDREW'S AMBULANCE ASSOCIATION ST JOHN AMBULANCE

The First Aid Manual

▶▶ sportscotland

For the latest publications please see: www.sportscotland.org.uk

▶▶ ROYAL LIFE SAVING SOCIETY (RLSS)

Books:
  Lifesaving
  Life Support
  Swim, Survive, Save

▶▶ BRITISH ASSOCIATION OF SKI PATROLLERS

Manual and Workbook:
  Outdoor First Aid and Safety

FURTHER COURSES

▶▶ BRITISH RED CROSS ST ANDREW'S AMBULANCE ASSOCIATION ST JOHN AMBULANCE

First Aid Course

▶▶ NATIONAL OUTDOOR TRAINING CENTRES

Glenmore Lodge (Scotland)
Plas y Brenin (Wales)
Tollymore (Northern Ireland)
Plas Menai (Wales)

Selected courses on:
  Outdoor Safety and First Aid

▶▶ ROYAL LIFE SAVING SOCIETY (RLSS)

Courses on aspects of:
Lifesaving
Life Support
Open Water Rescue
Swimming Pool Rescue
Specialist Training
Training and Assessing

National Occupational Standards for Coaching, Teaching and Instructing

The National Occupational Standards for Coaching, Teaching and Instructing (NOS) are based around a number of competences associated with planning, delivering and evaluating coaching sessions and programmes. The standards are used as part of national governing bodies' coach education awards and as the definition of competence for Scottish/National Vocational Qualifications (S/NVQs) in coaching, teaching and instructing. S/NVQs at Levels 2 and 3 are available in a number of sports. **sports coach UK** has developed its Coach Development Programme around these standards. **sports coach UK** workshops and resources aim to provide the underpinning knowledge for coaches who wish to meet the competences of the standards. They also give coaches guidelines on how to apply this knowledge to their coaching practice.

The Coach Workshop Programme and its supporting resources have been developed around Level 3 NOS. This resource and its associated workshop, *Injury Prevention and Management* has been designed to support the following units of the Level 3 NOS:

Unit C310 Provide emergency aid

C310.1 Respond to situations where there are injuries or illnesses
C310.2 Provide emergency aid to unconscious casualties
C310.3 Provide emergency aid to casualties who are bleeding
C310.4 Hand casualties over to qualified assistance

Unit C35 Deal with accidents and emergencies

C35.1 Deal with injuries and signs of illness
C35.2 Follow emergency procedures

For further information on the National Occupational Standards for Coaching, Teaching and Instructing at Level 3, contact **sports coach UK** or SPRITO at the following addresses:

sports coach UK
114 Cardigan Road
Headingley
Leeds
LS6 3BJ

Tel: 0113-274 4802
Fax: 0113-275 5019

E-mail: coaching@sportscoachuk.org
Website: www.sportscoachuk.org

The National Training Organisation
  for Sport, Recreation and Allied
  Occupations (SPRITO)
24 Stephenson Way
London
NW1 2HD

Tel: 020-7388 7755
Fax: 020-7388 9733

E-mail: tcl@sprito.org.uk
Website: www.sprito-els.org.uk

Index

t

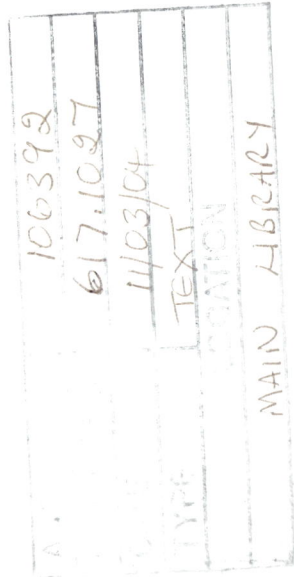